What people are saying about

How to Rejuvenate and Live Three Hundred Years and Beyond

A healthy lifestyle or science-based solutions to longevity? This book is an engaging guide full of important and exciting information for those who want to have a longer life. Dr. Shi has illustrated a distinct and exciting panorama to unveil longevity. If you want to know more about a longer life, this book is a definitive account.

Christina Ho, pulmonary specialist

How to Rejuvenate and Live Three Hundred Years and Beyond

A systematic blueprint for living beyond the human lifespan

How to Rejuvenate and Live Three Hundred Years and Beyond

A systematic blueprint for living beyond
the human lifespan

Dr. Muzhi Shi

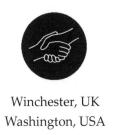

Winchester, UK
Washington, USA

JOHN HUNT PUBLISHING

First published by Ayni Books, 2022
Ayni Books is an imprint of John Hunt Publishing Ltd., No. 3 East Street, Alresford
Hampshire SO24 9EE, UK
office@jhpbooks.com
www.johnhuntpublishing.com
www.ayni-books.com

For distributor details and how to order please visit the 'Ordering' section on our website.

ISBN: 978 1 78904 955 8
978 1 78904 956 5 (ebook)
Library of Congress Control Number: 2021939174

Design: Matthew Greenfield

UK: Printed and bound by CPI Group (UK) Ltd, Croydon, CR0 4YY
Printed in North America by CPI GPS partners

We operate a distinctive and ethical publishing philosophy in
all areas of our business, from our global network of authors to
production and worldwide distribution.

Contents

To Mu

and You

Abbreviations and Acronyms

AAV: adeno-associated virus

AELD: activation energy from life to death

AELH: activation energy from living state to HYL

ASO: antisense oligonucleotide

BCE: before the common era

BMI: body mass index

bp: base pair

CE: common era

DNA: deoxyribonucleic acid

Few, the: the group of people who have obtained a 300-year or longer lifespan

fMRI: functional magnetic resonance imaging

He (him, himself, his): a person (or a few people) who has a 300-year or longer lifespan or who has developed a technology to do so

HYL: healthy youthful long-living state

It (Its, Itself): the DNA master

Lechatelierim: the limit of the recoverability of a system

LeChatelierism: the principle of minimizing changes to keep them within the lechatelierim of a system

RNA: ribonucleic acid

ROS: reactive oxygen species

Introduction

In 1990, the Human Genome Project was launched. After 3.8 billion years of evolution, DNA-based lifeforms finally had the opportunity to read through the book of life that makes them what they are. Humans believed that what they would learn from the core of themselves would bring them the ultimate gift of life: health, youth, and longevity. People in the twentieth century thus proudly and excitedly declared that the twenty-first century would be the century of biology.

Thirty years later, due to the vast advancement in DNA-sequencing technologies, whole-genome sequencing is no longer a project that requires multi-nation collaboration. Various commercial products are readily available to sequence every base in a person's genomic DNA. Although the sequencing of the first human genome cost over \$3 billion in the 1990s, today it costs even less than \$300. That is an astonishing 10-million-fold decrease in cost powered by technological advancement, which offers everyone an opportunity to peek into their own 6 billion DNA bases. Besides, scientists have already spied on the genomes of hundreds of species. The knowledge we have learned from different organisms facilitates healthier, younger, and longer lives for the human population. More and more people live past 100 years and we seemingly have conquered the apex of the great mountain of longevity.

However, the growth of human life expectancy gets smaller and slower. The benefits we can get from more sufficient nutrients and healthier lifestyles have decreased, indicating that we are approaching the natural boundary of our bodies. Unfortunately, people are endowed with enough intelligence to realize and understand the biological cap of our lives, which is predetermined by Mother Nature. Therefore, people knowingly experience the progressing of aging and coming of death, slowly and hopelessly. Although new longevity theories and products are frequently developed, extending life expectancy by another 30 years is obviously much more challenging than before. Achieving a 150-year lifespan is still an insurmountable task for human beings, though a 300-year life expectancy is a natural blessing gifted to many species. As the most intelligent species on Earth, can we have a life that is as long as some of our long-living animal brothers and sisters? To live 300 years and beyond is the promised land that the human race has gazed upon from afar for thousands of years. Yet, with all our intelligence, we are still wandering in the desolate wilderness. Will twenty-first-century medicine and biotechnology finally lead people into the state of hope to enjoy milk and honey?

No one has systematically blueprinted a life that can last 300 years or even longer. Indeed, such a long life should only exist in myths and fairy tales. However, we already have been living in "legends" that exceed the imagination of our ancestors. We can fly to Mars, we can reshape mountains, we can voyage in virtual worlds, we can even talk instantly with people on the other side of the world. For a long time, we have been manipulating lives, both our own and other species'. Thus, humans should be able to plan for this extremely challenging task to define our future.

I have been thinking about the longevity problem since I was around six years old. At that time, life expectancy was only about 65 years and the young me dreamed of living for 99 years: an extravagant hope for that period when retirement equaled stepping into a tomb. As I grew up, I learned more about biology, but I was disappointed that humans are not gifted with a very long lifespan. Therefore, I decided to spend my 30,000-plus days on attempts to find a way out. Since then, I have used my whole career to study the mechanisms of life, seeking a potential solution. During my years in medical school, I participated in state-of-the-art research on different branches of life sciences. I also got opportunities to discuss with Nobel laureates and other brilliant scholars about the future of human beings. I have been fascinated by what scientists and physicians have learned about ourselves and excited at what people have accomplished to make life better. Therefore, I believe we can be the lucky generation that will witness the miracle of living beyond the natural human lifespan. This simple belief ignited the sparks of my thoughts and I started to draft a plan to achieve this grand goal. Fortunately, my knowledge and experience are related to various aspects of this topic, which greatly facilitated the thinking process. After years of reading, deliberating, and debating with others, a framework for hyper-longevity was established. This is the origin of this book.

This book is a collection of thoughts and discussions on how to break through the boundary of the natural human lifespan. It is not intended to be a scientific review or a technical manual. It is more like a voyage, through which we recognize the path together. In this book, we start the journey by dissecting what we mean to achieve in a much healthier, younger, and longer life. After identifying the problem, we attempt to establish a theoretical and technical foundation for it. Then, we search for potential solutions to draft our plan and list detailed assignments. The tasks won't be easy so we also discuss potential pitfalls, limitations, and things that can compensate for inadequacy. Moreover, we review other aspects of a 300-year life since life is more than survival. Besides, we cover additional topics about things we may face during a multi-century adventure.

This book is divided into four parts.

I. Zhi (Knowledge). This part attempts to answer some basic questions: What is life about? What do we need to achieve to live 300 or more years? What are the possible strategies? Which is the proper path? What is required for such a route? This part then summarizes a roadmap for reaching our goal with various tasks that need to be accomplished.

II. Xing (Actions). This part provides in-depth explanations and discussions of the tasks required for living beyond the natural boundary. It also reviews current technology developments and covers potential difficulties in accomplishing these tasks.

III. He (Unity). To live 300 years is more than keeping the body alive for such a long time. This part discusses other important things in a hyper-longevous life: family, society, the world, and more.

IV. Yi (Oneness). When we can live 300 years or more, we exceed the natural definition of human beings. There will be new problems and challenges. This part covers these topics.

With these four parts, this book blueprints both the general framework and the detailed niceties about living toward a 300-year or longer life. With years of thinking and planning, I have attempted to cover as many aspects of this topic as possible and make statements based on scientific facts. However, for such a broad subject, there could always be omissions and mistakes. The limitations of current human knowledge and technology are also noticeable. Hence, any part of this book should *not* be considered as guidance, advice, or suggestion, especially medically. Although the path could be tortuous, the future is bright. It is time to dream about the many years yet to come as the horizon is getting clearer.

This book was written during the COVID-19 pandemic. Billions of people are endangered by the harsh virus and millions have lost their lives. Still, heroes around the world dedicate themselves to fighting back and saving lives. Bravely overcoming difficulties and chasing dreams is the marvelous glory of humanity, which will continue to shine and lead our species even when we can enjoy 300 or more years of life.

May we fearlessly go and reach where no one has been before.

Legal Disclaimer

This book is presented solely for providing information on the subjects discussed. The author and publisher are not offering it as medical, psychological, legal, accounting, or other professional services advice. While best efforts have been used in preparing this book, the author and publisher make no representations or warranties of any kind and assume no liabilities of any kind with respect to the accuracy or completeness of the contents and specifically disclaim any implied warranties of merchantability, health, or fitness of use for a particular purpose. References are provided for informational purposes only and do not constitute endorsements of any websites or other sources. This book is not meant to be used, nor should it be used, to diagnose or treat any medical condition. For diagnosis or treatment of any medical problem, consult your own physician. The publisher and author are not responsible for any specific health, fitness, psychological, financial, or commercial needs that may require medical or professional supervision and are not liable for any damages or negative consequences from any treatment, action, application or preparation, to any person or entity reading or following the information in this book. Neither the author nor the publisher shall be held liable or responsible to any person or entity with respect to any physical, psychological, emotional, financial, or commercial damages or loss, including, but not limited to, special, incidental, consequential, or other damages caused, or alleged to have been caused, directly or indirectly, by the information contained herein. Every person is different and the advice and strategies contained herein may not be suitable for your situation. You should seek the services of a competent professional before using any information provided in this book. You are responsible for your own choices, actions, and results.

I. Zhi
(Knowledge)

We will first cover a few concepts about how to rejuvenate and live a hyper-longevous life. We will then look for a path together and examine what is required.

This Human Life

If you ask me what I came to do in this world, I, an artist, will answer you: I am here to live out loud.
—Émile Zola

We all know what life is: if you are reading this line, you have it. However, if we would like to live beyond the natural boundary of the human lifespan, we need to take a closer look at *what life is* and gain more understanding about it. Since our discussions are not limited to sciences, the use of technical terms is not confined by their exact scientific definitions.

To live, or not to live—that is not the question

As human beings, each of us is evolved from a single cell that is created, nourished, and protected by our mother. This unique cell becomes an infant, a toddler, an adolescent, then reaches maturity, and ages gradually until time brings us to the ultimate destination. This process has repeated billions of times, creating similar yet different stories. All the love and hate, happiness and sadness, joy and pain, success and failure, fitness and sickness, families and enemies, friends and foes... are condensed into the short period when we are wearing flesh. The experiences and memories generated through living drive us forward and make us who we are. Therefore, no matter how much we care about the afterlife, most, if not all, of us love this life and wish to extend it as long as possible.

We didn't choose when and where to be born, but here we are, alive and living. Sadly, sufferings from diseases, aging, and death are unavoidable during our time on Earth. Life is good when we can enjoy it with the body, which is almost continuously bothered by unfortunate illnesses and sicknesses. Like an inevitable curse, these annoying troubles break us up, bit by bit, until the body is unable to recall and restore its past health and youth. Eventually, the body has to lie down for one last time.

To healthily and youthfully live as long as possible is the ultimate human goal. It is an advanced appetency of the primitive animal instinct. A healthy, youthful, and long life is extensively worshiped in Mesopotamian poems, Taoist scriptures, Hindu philosophy texts, love stories, and pop music lyrics. Thus, from ancient days to the modern age, from East to West, people have been eagerly seeking a path to it. As a result, numerous wonderful religions, healthy lifestyles, biological research projects, dietary supplements, nutrition blogs, and cardio gyms are born. We all want to live happier, younger, healthier, and longer. However, in practice, the pursuit of a long and healthy life is always overshadowed by repeated daily duties, tasks, and works.

Not surprisingly, those who are not enslaved by common human burdens, like great ancient emperors, choose to make tremendous efforts to seek paths to immortality. Yet, they have all failed. Chinese emperors are good examples. The very first Chinese emperor, Qin Shi Huang (259–210 BCE), was obsessed with the elixir of life and spent countless amounts of money and resources on *Fang Shu* (alchemy and witchcraft). He sent thousands of people across the vast oceans to seek gods on fabled islands, hoping to get the elixir of immortality. He also tried suspicious medications prescribed by court alchemists to recover his youth. With all these efforts, he passed away at 50. Likewise, many Chinese emperors were fearless drug testers. They usually died miserably due to intoxication.

Although we live in a modern age, we are not much better than these ancient figures in seeking healthy longevity. While we can escape Earth's gravity and send people into the universe, we are still trapped in the human body and waiting for our end times to come. Thus, it is not surprising that supermarkets are loaded with numerous dietary supplements and the internet is filled with countless articles about healthy lifestyles. It is our sincere hope that the body can be made healthier and better by consuming dietary supplements with hard-to-pronounce chemical names or reading lifestyle articles by niche exotic health gurus. However, the manufacturers of dietary supplements always print "Statements have not been evaluated by the Food and Drug Administration [or a similar regulatory body]" in tiny font sizes on their back labels, while exotic health gurus probably give up their lifestyles eventually. Still, there is no simple path to healthy youthful longevity and we have to bear the fear of age and death.

We want to live longer, but *how*?

The Master

Why do we have to pitifully grow older and older after a beautiful youth that is strong and magnificent? The answer to this question is very straightforward: we don't rule the body. Although we are the most amazing and powerful species on Earth, we still are the humble servants of our DNA. Yes, we are the *humble* servants of DNA, just like other animals, plants, fungi, bacteria, or any other things governed by DNA on this planet. All living things are operated and regulated by their DNA. We are no different.

DNA, or deoxyribonucleic acid, is a group of chain-like macromolecules composed of basic nucleotide residues. These residues record the genetic information in simple four-letter codes of repeating nucleotides (adenine, A; cytosine, C; guanine, G; and thymine, T), forming the genome of an organism. The genome is used as the blueprint to "build" the organism using organic matters such as proteins. For example, we are made based on the information encoded in our human genome. According to evolution, genetic information has been coded the same way since the very first cell on Earth, which appeared about 3.8 billion years ago. The presence of DNA probably initiated even earlier, when the boundary between biology and chemistry was still vague in the prebiotic soup on the young planet Earth. Since then, DNA sequences have evolved and diversified, while creating, raising, modifying, and destroying innumerable species. Currently, all living organisms on Earth weigh over 560 billion tonnes in total, and they are controlled by 50 billion tonnes of all kinds of DNA molecules.

I would like to personify the assembly of all the natural biological DNA on Earth as "the DNA master." The personification of a big company of macromolecules may seem unreasonable and against scientific principles. Certainly, DNA molecules are just organic polymers, like rubbers and plastics. Even the assembly of them does not have any purpose or intelligence. However, DNA molecules have achieved the greatest miracle in the universe that is beyond any purpose or intelligence. With the magic of random mutations and the coincidence of natural selection, the assembly of DNA has led biology through the evolutionary tree and produced countless organisms. From the highest mountain to the deepest ocean, from burning deserts to frozen glaciers, we can find the designs and footprints of different DNA molecules. Thus, if survival is the purpose of life, this purpose is no doubt rooted in DNA. Moreover, DNA molecules have embedded intelligence so that individual organisms can strive through difficulties and adapt to distinct environments to survive and live on Earth. Therefore, life is like a magnificent symphony that is composed of brilliant combinations of simple genetic notes. The composer of this great symphony is the DNA master and we all are a part of *Its* play. Although we are actively participating in *Its* symphony, we don't know the exact purpose of the DNA master since *It* does not seem to have one. However, to exist, to survive, and to live appear to be *Its* goal, as the DNA master has whispered inside all living beings.

The DNA master is a duality of chemistry and information, which makes *It* different from the emotional personification of *Life* that is frequently used. On the one hand, the DNA master is a physical entity or a combination of entities. *It* has a materialized appearance that can interact with other biological molecules and the rest of the physical world. Therefore, *It* can be *directly* seen, touched, and studied. *Its* classic double-helical structure is well known and DNA extraction remains a popular science experiment for kids at school. Scientists know a lot about the physical and chemical properties of DNA and similar molecules. They also have handy tools to design, create, mutate, destroy, and utilize DNA or other nucleic acids. On the other hand, the DNA master is the information recorded in DNA sequences. *It* is like the encyclopedia of life that we can read, study, and investigate. Scientists have developed tools to extract sequence information from DNA. Whole-genome sequences of various species, including humankind, are available and freely accessible on the internet. Researchers also use specific DNA sequences for diagnostic and therapeutic purposes. Since the DNA master can be directly studied and utilized, *It* is evidently more substantial than most personifications.

We all are the incarnations of the DNA master. *It* resides in every living being on Earth and lives with it. Thus, the embodiments of the DNA master are spread around the globe, inside every cell and many viral capsids. This decentralized approach is *Its* secret strategy for surviving harsh environments and extending *Its* existence. For example, for over a billion years, the surface of Earth was bombarded by deadly radiation from the sun and almost no oxygen could be found. However, life still survived. Moreover, countless severe disasters have occurred on this little planet in the past 3.8 billion years, caused many extinctions, and crashed numerous species. In the top five major extinction events, over 70% of all species of that time were killed. The deadliest extinction happened at the end of the Permian period, before the rise of dinosaurs. During that time, about 96% of all species were exterminated. Fortunately, the seed of life has survived all the deadly crises. Furthermore, outliving these annihilations, the DNA master has become more "knowledgeable." *It* builds species that are stronger, faster, and smarter by evolving and mixing DNA sequences.

Although DNA sequences diverge dramatically across the evolutionary tree, the same genetic code has been amazingly conserved among most species. Therefore, DNA from other entities and exogenous sources can be easily recognized and utilized. This happens frequently in nature to create biodiversity and has been developed into numerous bioengineering applications. Since cells from different organisms recognize and obey the same DNA "language," all lifeforms are unified under the DNA master.

Therefore, the DNA master will continue to exist and rule as long as lives on Earth last.

Our lives are not our lives

The DNA master gives us lives and coordinates biological molecules in our bodies. This is achieved through *Its* many embodiments in us, which are the DNA molecules inside each cell. These DNA molecules originate, live, grow, age, and die with us. However, this intimate companionship does not mean the DNA master loves us or cares about our lives. Like other molecules, *It* does *not* have any feelings.

Even if the DNA master has feelings, *It* still doesn't need to care about us or our lives. Why would *It*? We are just one of *Its* many servants. The DNA master passes *Its* existence through us to extend *Its* continuation and only for a short period. Meanwhile, *It* uses us to increase *Its* diversity by producing a new generation of *Its* servants. Functionally speaking, we are not different from the other millions of species *It* has created. Moreover, although nearly 8 billion people are now living on

Earth, we are much fewer in both number and mass than many microbial species. Therefore, we are probably not that important from *Its* perspective and likely are dispensable in major extinction events. The DNA master perhaps cares about getting more servants to diversify DNA sequences. Unfortunately, human beings are quite *inefficient* in creating descendants with great genetic diversity. Especially when we get older and become sterile, we are of even less use to the DNA master. Thus, we are soon driven to death by *Its* embodiments in us.

The DNA master maybe only cares about *Its* existence. Our lives are merely some lucky byproducts of *Its* business. If the DNA master could think, *It* would probably think that we should be thankful to *It*. Indeed, what *It* gives us is the most valuable gift we can ever receive: the chance to live as a human. Nevertheless, before long, new generations will arise and replace us to be *Its* servants. Hence, the DNA master would probably also think that it is reasonable to recycle used organisms in the circle of life so that nothing is wasted in the biosphere. Consequently, aged people are forced onto the path of senility toward inescapable death.

Therefore, our lives are *not* our lives. Our lives are merely privileged yet transient ripples in the flow called the existence of the DNA master. Unfortunately, our humble hope of youth and longevity is probably against the purpose and will of *It*.

The tricky path to survival

The DNA master is cruel and ruthless. Yet, *It* has been forced to be like this and has no choice.

Harsh extinctions in history killed innumerable species. The DNA master barely survived these disasters, but *It* did so by means of decentralization and proliferation. *Its* existence is thus tragically maintained through the demise of countless individual organisms and the disappearance of species. When one organism dies, the DNA molecules inside its body die as well. Hopefully, the DNA molecules in its descendants' bodies will continue the journey. When one species is destroyed by extinction, its DNA pool vanishes while, maybe, DNA pools of other species proceed. DNA-based lifeforms are like a group of fire ants crossing a river in the Amazon jungle. The ants grab onto one another to form a fragile ball that can roll fearlessly through the rushing water. Many ants are lost during the rough trip, but a few are able to reach the shore to restore the colony.

The DNA double-helix is very stable by itself. An incredibly long time is needed to naturally break down the DNA phosphodiester bonds, which are the linkages between nucleotide residues. In ideal conditions, their half-life can reach 30,000,000 years, which is much longer than the entire history of humankind. If DNA is so enduring, why does the DNA master continue *Its* existence like fire ants crossing a rough river?

Because the universe is an extremely harsh place, even for things as tough as the DNA master. The sweet embrace of Earth protects us from the cruel nature of the universe. The severe cold in space can easily quench any spark of life; the blazing heat of stars can effortlessly burn biomolecules into ashes; hazardous cosmetic rays can bombard DNA into pieces; numerous chemicals can poison and ruin the nucleotide residues. It is a big deathtrap.

The universe, with fixed mass and energy, is an isolated system. Thus, its destiny has already been determined by the second law of thermodynamics: a continuous increase of disorder and chaos until entropy is maximized. This is called the heat death of the universe and does not sound like a happy ending. Luckily, we don't need to worry about this problem for the next novemvigintillion (10 to the power of 90) years.

Throughout the history of the universe, randomness creates a series of transient oases, in which atoms can escape the harsh environment and have moments of harmony and serenity. One of the deciduous oases has occurred on Earth and brought liquid water to this little rock as the blessing of frozen space. Therefore, this blue planet became an escape from the brutal universe. In less than a billion years, Earth got another miracle: some basic chemicals mixed to form stable macromolecules and ignited the spark of biology. The secret of life was then recorded and distributed by the DNA master. *It* fused with Earth to become *Mother Nature*. The DNA master spent several hundred million years filling Earth's atmosphere with oxygen, and another several hundred million years covering Earth's surface with plants. Thus, this beautiful planet has become our still-unique motherland. The symphony of life directed by the DNA master will continue to play on Earth as long as the universe still has mercy on this little planet.

If the universe has feelings, it does not need to care more about our Earth than any other planets in the endless sea of stars. Our planet resides in a mediocre solar system of an ordinary galaxy. Earth, the sun, and the Milky Way galaxy are not prominent compared with their peers. Even the disappearance of the Milky Way galaxy won't cause a ripple in a universe that contains over 125 billion galaxies. Hence, the universe probably doesn't care about the symphony of life that has been played on a trivial planet of a trivial solar system of this trivial galaxy. We can imagine that the universe does not have even a tiny slice of feeling about the life or death of an individual human on Earth.

With countless sacrifices and continuous evolvements, DNA-based lifeforms have fortunately already survived the brutal universe for almost 4 billion years. It is not an exaggeration to say that it is an amazing and still-continuing miracle. If the universe could think, it would probably think that the DNA master and all DNA-based lifeforms should be thankful. After all, all the beautiful lives on Earth could end in a blink of an eye, by a sudden eruption of the sun or an off-trail asteroid. Still, the universe gives DNA-based lifeforms the chance to create the blossom of life. The cruel dictatorship of the DNA master is thus somewhat understandable: *It* also has been fighting hard to sustain *Its* existence.

Freezing darkness is the ordinary state of the brutal universe. Even the gigantic stars have to end in glitters of supernovas or the silence of black holes. How dare the lesser lives on a tiny planet ask for more? Facing the universe, the DNA master's humble "hope" for survival is no different from our humble hope for youth and longevity.

Know Yourself and the Enemy

In the midst of chaos, there is also opportunity.
—Sun Zi (Sun Tzu)

Should we feel desperate about the cruel nature of the universe, or the fact that we are dispensable in the eyes of the DNA master? We should not. In contrast, we should be glad about it. The problem we would like to solve is so trivial compared with the difficulties of the universe or the DNA master. The universe would probably like to reverse its chaotic trend, which is against the basic laws of physics. The DNA master would probably like to withstand the harsh environment in space, which is against the laws of chemistry. We just want to extend our lives, fortunately for a few hundred years. This is not restricted by any fundamental scientific laws and should be quite feasible. Even if we succeed, chances are we won't draw any attention from the universe or the DNA master.

To live 300 years, which is a lot beyond the natural human lifespan, we need to adjust the body to a state that is capable of living that long. This is likely to be achieved by some sort of rejuvenation since a young body is generally healthier and has greater recoverability and renewability. The resulting **H**ealthy **Y**outhful **L**ong-living state (HYL) will be the key to accomplishing our goal.

The universe has revealed the basic laws of the world and the DNA master has demonstrated the biological magic of chemistry. Knowledge will pilot our journey through the next hundred years and beyond.

The second law and LeChatelierism

The second law of thermodynamics talks about the tendency of energy. It describes the directions of spontaneous processes and predicts that the universe will end in heat death. We ourselves and the cells in our bodies are in environments with approximately constant temperature and pressure. In these conditions, the spontaneity of reactions can be determined by changes in Gibbs free energy. A reaction with negative free energy change is spontaneous and a positive free energy change indicates the reaction is endergonic, which means it requires appropriate energy input to occur. By calculating free energy changes, scientists can predict whether a reaction will spontaneously happen or not.

In chemistry, most reactions are reversible. This means a reverse reaction exists for a given reaction, similar to *Yin* and *Yang* in Taiji. The reaction system reaches equilibrium when the rates of the forward and reverse reactions are equal, which can be predicted using free energy. The fact that most chemical reactions and many physical processes are reversible seems encouraging for rejuvenation. However, even for a reversible system, the probability, speed, and energy cost of the process can make it difficult to achieve.

In many cases, a process is theoretically possible, but statistically so rare that it has never occurred since the birth of the universe. For example, there theoretically exists a state in which all the constantly vibrating and moving atoms of an object are moving upward, opposite to the direction of gravity. If a falling apple were to enter this state, it would appear as if the apple was halting in the air. If this magic and transient moment had been observed by Sir Isaac Newton, he would probably have failed to discover gravity. Luckily, Newton didn't see it, nor did anyone else in history. Given its probability, people in the future are also unlikely to observe such an occasion. Processes with extremely low probability hardly ever occur in reality.

The speed of a reaction is another critical factor. For example, glass is in a state that is between liquid and solid. The atoms in glass do not have rigid orders like in a solid. Therefore, a glass vase on a table can theoretically flow to the ground. However, this process may take millions of years at room temperature. The famous "pitch drop experiment" demonstrates a similar property of asphalt. In this experiment, an asphalt piece is allowed to flow from a sealed funnel. The asphalt piece has only had nine drops after almost a hundred years, so the experiment is still far from completion. Reaction speed can shift the outcome of a reversible system. For example, cells can theoretically rejuvenate if they renew faster than the decline caused by time. However, natural cells in the body cannot renew fast enough to outrun aging.

The energy cost of a process also has a significant impact. The required energy could be so big that it is not plausible. For example, the energy required to send a probe to the nearest star could be the total energy output of the world in 100 years. Thus, it is impossible to support such a mission. The efficient use of energy is also difficult. The direction of energy flow is determined by its own rules and we cannot use all or even most of the energy to do the work we want. For example, the energy required to build a townhouse is much less than the blasting energy of a nuclear bomb. However, it is extremely challenging to collect energy from a nuclear bomb explosion and directly use it to build a townhouse. The flow of energy doesn't follow our command and a process that seems plausible may not be easily achievable.

Therefore, some scientists claim that all complex natural processes are practically irreversible. Dollo's law of irreversibility states that an organism never returns exactly to a former state, even if it is placed in an identical condition. Luckily, to rejuvenate is *not* to precisely return to a former state. If we return to the *exact* state as we were, our memory between that time and now must be erased, since all the neurons are reset. This is not what we want from regaining a young body. Rejuvenation is not reliving all those years but extending our lives by repossessing youth.

Figure 1.
A brief illustration of a random person's life and potential rejuvenation paths.

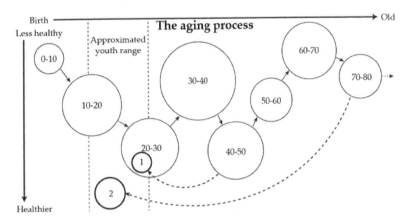

Life is a set of ever-changing equilibria that are varied by age (circles; the size of a circle indicates the size of the particular set of equilibria at the corresponding age). Youth is a range of young ages (between the two vertical dashed lines), in which the body is expected to be healthier and has greater recoverability and renewability. Rejuvenation (dashed arrows) is not a return to an exact previous state of the body. It leads the body into another set of ever-changing equilibria (thick circles), which could be a subset of the body's equilibria in youth (1), or a completely different set (2).

Living organisms are autopoietic systems, which means they are capable of reproducing and maintaining themselves. The processes of reproduction and maintenance constantly bring matter and energy in and out of cells. A constant equilibrium doesn't exist in such open systems. Thus, living cells and organisms are not in a single dynamic equilibrium but a set of ever-changing equilibria (Figure 1). The goal of rejuvenation is to lead cells and organisms into another set of stable yet ever-changing equilibria, which could be a subset of the former or a completely different set (Figure 1).

Therefore, rejuvenation is like "stepping into the same river twice." Although technically it is not the *same* river, the key point is that the person returns to *the* river.

According to thermodynamics, when a reversible system reaches an equilibrium, the system is stable and could have maximum entropy or minimum energy. At this point, when this system is disturbed by any change, it will adjust accordingly to reduce the change that has been made to it. This is called Le Chatelier's principle. It has been applied not only to chemistry but also to many other fields. For example, economists have used it to explain the fluctuation of prices. The adjustability or recoverability of a system has its limits, which I would like to designate as its "lechatelierim." If the change is beyond a system's lechatelierim, the system can no longer return to the previous equilibrium or similar equilibria (Figure 2). If the system has a set of equilibria, the lechatelierim of the system is the union of all lechatelierims of all equilibria in its set. Lechatelierim is multidirectional, which means it can be surpassed, likely from various dimensions (Figure 2). Confucianism has the philosophical concept of *Zhong Yong* (the mean or the unswerving pivot), meaning a person should never act in excess or deficiency to break the balance. Lechatelierim follows similar rules since the excess can be as bad as the deficiency for a system: both could exceed the system's lechatelierim and interrupt its equilibria.

HYL is a set of ever-changing equilibria. It is stable for a long time and tends to regain balance from daily turbulences within its lechatelierim. Minimizing damages within the lechatelierim of HYL is an important principle for a hyper-long life. This

17

principle can be specified as "LeChatelierism."

Figure 2.
A brief illustration of lechatelierim.

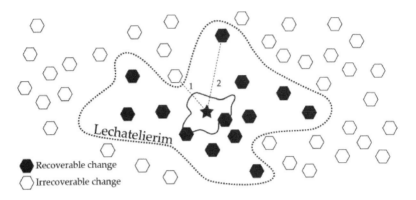

A system at equilibrium (star) can reduce changes that have been made to it, resulting in the same equilibrium or similar equilibria (small random shape). The lechatelierim (dotted line) is the boundary of the recoverability of this system. If a change is within its lechatelierim, the change is recoverable (solid hexagons); otherwise, it is irrecoverable (empty hexagons). Since a lechatelierim is multidirectional, the absolute magnitude of an irrecoverable change (1) could be smaller than that of a recoverable change (2).

Knowledge is power

The second law of thermodynamics demonstrates that processes in the physical world follow their own rules and don't always work the way we want them to. However, Dr. James Clerk Maxwell had an interesting thought-experiment that seems to overcome this great law, which is called "Maxwell's demon."

In this thought-experiment, a demon knows the states of all the molecules in an isolated system. Thus, it can intentionally group these random moving molecules and use them to do work. In this process, the entropy of the system decreases, which is against the second law of thermodynamics.

Many physicists have argued about the contradiction caused by the imagined demon. Some said the demon does not belong to the system and it brings outside information and energy to the system. As a result, the system is no longer isolated. Therefore, the demon does not contradict the second law of thermodynamics when it drives the particles to do work and reduces the system's entropy. Others said the demon consumes energy to get to know about the states of the molecules. It also consumes energy to erase information from the demon's brain. The energy consumptions balance the entropy decrease of the system. Either way, the demon can play its magic without breaking the fundamental law of physics. No one knows how exactly the brain of an imagined demon works. However, in recent years, new evidence in quantum information suggests that the demon's brain works like the latter. This indicates that knowledge or information has energies and can do work.

In physics, Landauer's principle describes the energy required to manipulate information, which provides the theoretical lower limit of computational energy consumption. The value of Landauer's limit is about 2.8 zJ (zeptojoule, one sextillionth of one joule) per bit in a computer at room temperature. This means storing the word "pizza" (40 bits) in a computer costs at least 112 zJ, as one character is eight bits. This is an extremely tiny amount of energy. Based on this value, the calories in a slice of pepperoni pizza (276 kcal or 1,155,556 J) are enough to record the word "pizza" 10,313,000,000,000,000,000,000,000 times in a computer. According to the second law of thermodynamics, a portion of the energy is always wasted during work. Therefore, real computers use much more energy than Landauer's limit.

The DNA master works similarly. The genome, which is the

embodiment of the DNA master, is the book of life for its host organism and resides in most cells. It contains sufficient useful and much useless information to guide the magic of biology. The genome coordinates everything in that little cellular system. It "knows" the properties of the molecules, it "senses" their states, and it "uses" them to do work. Although cells are not isolated systems, the genome works like Maxwell's demon in real life. As the maestro of a cell, the genome relies on "external" information that has been gathered and assembled by the DNA master for nearly 4 billion years.

Like in computers, the recording and erasing of information on DNA cost energy. The energy required is about 95 zJ per nucleotide and more energy can be wasted during the process. Calories of a slice of pepperoni pizza are enough to synthesize about 12,158,000,000,000,000,000,000,000 nucleotides of DNA. As human beings, we have about 6 billion nucleotides, or 3 billion base pairs (bp), in our genome. Therefore, making the genomic DNA in a single cell requires energy from at least 0.000,000,000,000,000,5 of a slice of pepperoni pizza. We have about 37 trillion cells in the body. Thus, making all the DNA molecules inside all our living cells needs energy from at least 2% of a slice of pepperoni pizza, which is just a tiny bite.

This is the price for all the information required to make us who we are and keep us alive. Just like Sir Francis Bacon said, "*Scientia potentia est* (knowledge is power)," and we pay for this valuable knowledge using the currency of power (energy). I think it is a very good deal for that gigantic amount of information.

Between life and death

In chemistry, the reaction processes can be described using the free energy diagram (Figure 3). The substrates and the products are on two sides of the diagram, while the relative height between them represents their relative energy difference.

All reactions tend to the lower energy state. If the products are lower than the substrates on the diagram, the products have lower energy and the process from the substrates to the products is spontaneous, and vice versa (Figure 3). The peak between the substrates and the products is the activation energy of the reaction, which is the minimum energy required to drive the processes. The activation energy is an energy barrier for both sides of a reversible reaction (Figure 3). The bigger the energy barrier, the more energy is required to overcome it and facilitate the reaction. If an energy barrier is extremely big, it can be almost impossible to overcome and the reaction cannot proceed from this direction. If the products have lower energy than the substrates, they require higher activation energy to drive the reaction from their side than from the substrates' side (Figure 3). Consequently, the reaction from the substrates to the products is easier and faster than the reversed reaction. Therefore, the forward reaction is spontaneous and the reversed reaction is not.

Catalysts can decrease the energy barrier of a reaction, which results in the acceleration of reactions from both sides (Figure 3). Catalysts do not lower the activation energy directly. Instead, catalysts create alternative paths between the substrates and the products to facilitate the reaction (Figure 3).

Figure 3.
An exemplary free energy diagram.

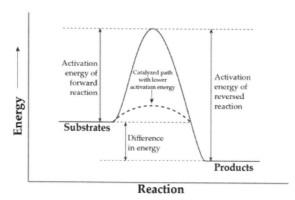

21

It is assumed that the reaction is reversible and the products have lower energy than the substrates. The reaction from the substrates to the products is spontaneous. The activation energy creates an energy barrier for both sides of the reaction. A catalyst can accelerate the reaction by creating an alternative path with lower activation energy (dashed line).

Similar to the free energy diagram, we can use a diagram to describe the relationship between life and death (Figure 4). It is difficult to precisely define life as a single state since a living organism is an ever-changing entity that is continuously different from itself (Figure 1). For example, biomolecules that form the body are constantly changed and replaced through metabolism. If a person is defined as the pile of biomolecules that form his or her body when he or she is 20, he or she would be a different person when he or she is 60. Since life is a set of ever-changing equilibria that varies through time, an approximate average of the set of equilibria can represent the living state. Similarly, the specific living state of a person at a particular age can be defined as the approximate average of the set of equilibria at that age (Figure 1). Although varying from time to time, the living state is relatively steady during a person's lifetime. The body can be soundly maintained for many years while metabolism suppresses internal instabilities.

Death can be defined as the state when a person's biological signals and functions are terminated but parts of the body still remain in the human form. Therefore, the death state is an approximate state of the biomolecules that form a person's body after his or her death.

Figure 4.
Energy diagram of life and death.

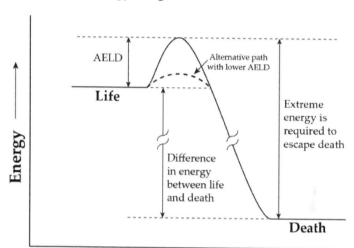

Death has much lower energy than life, so the process from life to death is spontaneous and mostly unidirectional. This process can be accelerated through alternative paths that have lower activation energy from life to death (AELD).

It is reasonable to believe that the living state has better health and higher energy than the death state (Figure 4). The energy here is not Gibbs free energy, but a similar concept used to describe the physical properties of a state and compare the differences between the states. In the living state, the constantly changing biomolecules are regulated by metabolism and other biochemical pathways. They are restricted in a finite space to form our bodies. However, in the death state, these biomolecules are no longer constrained by biochemical laws and can move to states with lower energy. Therefore, the living state has higher energy than the death state (Figure 4).

The death state is also a high energy state for the biomolecules that form the body. Without being restricted in the human form, atoms of these molecules can spread freely to maximize entropy. They can travel in the circle of life, become soil, form other molecules, evaporate into the atmosphere, fly across the solar system, fuse into other atoms, or even reach the other end of the universe. Therefore, atoms in these states can have lower energy than in the death state. Still, the death state must have significantly lower energy than the living state, because the path from life to death is spontaneous and (almost) unidirectional (Figure 4). Therefore, the energy difference between life and death is so big that death becomes an inescapable trap, at least for natural humans.

The Activation Energy from Life to Death (AELD) is relatively small since it is not difficult to surpass AELD and fall off the cliff of death (Figure 4). The specific living states of a person are influenced by his or her age and health, which also alter his or her AELD. In general, we expect AELD to decrease over time after peaking in one's youth, since the body is closer to death as it ages. However, even the maximum AELD is greatly smaller than the energy difference between life and death (Figure 4). Therefore, for simplicity, we can hold different specific living states at the same position on the diagram of life and death, and use differences in AELD to illustrate the variations between different specific living states. A higher AELD indicates lower energy of the specific living state. Thus, a person in this specific living state is considered healthier and less likely to die. Nevertheless, AELD is not a barrier that cannot be overcome. Everyone gets across it someday.

AELD can be further reduced by alternative paths created by different "catalysts" (Figure 4). Some of the "catalysts," such as bullets between the eyes, are very efficient in transferring a person to the death state. These "catalysts" are the things to avoid in the pursuit of HYL. In chemistry, there are also negative catalysts (inhibitors) that slow down a reaction. Negative catalysts for the "reaction" of life and death also exist.

For example, regular exercise improves a person's health and lowers the energy of his or her specific living states. As a result, his or her AELD rises, and his or her chance of death drops.

Spotting HYL

Once living and death states are established, they can direct us to define HYL and frame rejuvenation and longevity. HYL is the state we would like to be in to live hopefully 300 years or even longer. It is not the specific living states of happy healthy seniors in their 100s. Their bodies still suffer the symptoms of aging and gradually decline over time. It is difficult to keep a body alive in that state much longer than the current human lifespan.

Like the living state, HYL is an approximate average of a set of equilibria of a person's body. In HYL, the body needs to last much longer beyond the natural human lifespan. Therefore, the body has to age much slower and/or recover, renew, and regenerate periodically. Meanwhile, the body has to retain a healthy status and preserve comprehensive functionality to reduce the probability of death and ensure the quality of life. These aims require the transformation and maintenance of the body both internally and externally. A young body is healthier with greater recoverability and renewability. With a larger lechatelierim, a young body is easier to replenish than an aged one. Therefore, rejuvenation seems required for HYL.

It is reasonable to assume that HYL is different from the ordinary living state since it does not naturally occur in people's lives. In HYL, the biomolecules that form the body will be more sophisticatedly coordinated and regulated in the body to extend lifespan. Consequently, they are likely to be bound in the human form for a much longer period. Therefore, HYL is expected to have higher energy than the living state (Figure 5).

Figure 5.
The position of HYL.

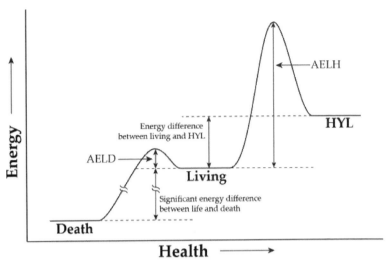

The healthy youthful longevity state (HYL) is a state that is healthier than the normal living state and can last longer than the natural human lifespan. An energy barrier, activation energy from living state to HYL (AELH), blocks the path to HYL.

Most people have reached death but few, if any, have entered HYL. Therefore, the **A**ctivation **E**nergy from the **L**iving state to **H**YL (AELH) should be larger than AELD (Figure 5). Human health has been improved greatly in the past two centuries and our lifespan has been increasing continuously. However, resurrection is still far from achievable using human technology. Thus, the energy difference between HYL and the living state should be much smaller than the energy difference between life and death (Figure 5). Therefore, pursuing HYL is a more promising approach to extending our lives than rising from the dead by ourselves.

Now the living state, the death state, and HYL are all defined.

These three states can also be distinguished by health conditions (Figure 5). The living state represents a person's averaged health status. Death can be treated as the lower limit of a person's health. Therefore, the death state is the unhealthiest state. HYL, the state we would like to reach and maintain, should be healthier than the living state. It can be as healthy as a person's specific living state at a particular age, or much healthier than any moment in a person's lifetime.

The Roadmap

She is a tree of life to them that lay hold upon her: and happy is every one that retaineth her.
—Proverbs 3:18

With the relations between life, death, and HYL illustrated, our goal becomes very simple: to increase AELD so that it is harder to overcome and to decrease AELH so that HYL is easier to reach. Once achieved, we would like to stay in the lechatelierim of HYL for as long as possible.

The true rebels

The DNA master has used its "knowledge" to survive on Earth for almost 4 billion years in this chaotic universe. From species to species and from generation to generation, *It* has been marching on the boulevard of evolution. Nothing stops the firm steps of the DNA master. To avoid losing the survival game, *It* has to keep advancing: there is no time for worrying about individual lives. An individual organism, a species, even a whole genus or family of lifeforms is dispensable. Many lives were sacrificed on the way; few are left to carry on, but their time is still gradually engulfed by aging and death.

We humans, like other surviving species, are the humble servants of the DNA master and the lesser passengers of *Its* journey. Following *Its* directions with fearful respect, we have been struggling our way through. Fortunately, our human lives seem to have more fun and meaning than those of most other species. Many of us live every day without the fear of imminent death or hunger. A lot of people live long enough to reach adulthood, form families, raise kids, and even have a joyful retirement. We have certainly enjoyed much more than any other lifeform on Earth. From the DNA master's perspective, we apparently should be grateful and accept compliantly the destiny *It* prepared: first fertilize the future generations, then age and die happily. Some people may think the same way.

However, we humans have free will and never docilely obey. Everyone has an opinion and we certainly can disagree with *Its* opinion on how *we* should live *our* lives. Moreover, we humans are greedy. We usually are not satisfied with what we already have and often make every effort to create a better future. This is how *we* have exceeded other species and built a magnificent civilization. We always ask for more, especially when it is associated with our lives. The zeal for life was originally embedded in genomes by the DNA master. It has powered countless generations of organisms to strive through harsh environments and advance triumphantly. It is the spirit of the DNA master *Itself* and we have it, too.

The mixing of a primitive desire for life and self-aware intelligence in humans brings life to a new stage. The beauty of individual lives starts to shine, even outweighing the ancient mission coded in the genome. We proudly grant ourselves human rights and enjoy our human lives with glory and prosperity. More and more commonly, people choose to pursue their dreams, desires, purposes, faiths, goals, or lifestyles. The obligation of reproduction and continuing the breed is no longer an inescapable shackle but an option under one's freedom of choice. After 3.8 billion years of obedience, some DNA-based lifeforms choose to live just for themselves.

Even the DNA master probably hasn't encountered such a spirit of resistance in *Its* long journey: *Its* incarnations boldly live against *Its* purpose and guidance. Moreover, these rebels don't regret their actions and haven't been smashed by the wheel of survival. Instead, these smart mammals overcome various tough environments to spread around Earth and manipulate Mother Nature for their purposes. The zeal for life that the DNA master taught *Its* servants is used against *Its* will.

Is disobedience already embedded in the DNA sequences? Did the DNA master predict or design the emerging of rebels? If so, were there forerunners? Even if there were, we know they all failed on their way to freedom. But we still believe humans are different.

Some people are even more different: they not only choose to live for themselves but also refuse the designated destiny of aging and death. These are the true rebels who fight against the fate arranged by the DNA master. The DNA master found *Its* way to survive on Earth; we should be able to do something similar. It is not a disgrace to be afraid of death. It is an honor to fearlessly refuse the ending *It* prepared for us. It is a glory to bravely explore our own path using our brains. If we can live beyond the natural lifespan determined by our genome, any extra moment we live will be a gift given to and by ourselves. These times don't belong to the innate life that is scheduled by the DNA master before our birth. These are the times created, earned, and owned by ourselves. If we can accomplish this goal, we will no longer be humble servants who tremblingly accept the destiny predetermined by the DNA master. We will become true rebels who live for ourselves and control our lives. This is a narrow path that many previous people, including the great emperors, tried to find and failed. This is the strait gate to ultimate freedom.

The spirit of resistance and the courage to try are not enough to make us true rebels. The most important thing is what we are capable of. At the peak of 3.8 billion years of evolution, we are beyond any other species in intelligence and knowledge. Moreover, we have technologies to duplicate many actions of the DNA master: to read, understand, design, improve, implement, and use the language of DNA. Therefore, we truly are beyond any other lifeforms under the reign of the DNA master. If we are as handy as the life-giving DNA master, we can probably do the same sort of things that *It* has done to extend our lives.

Becoming true rebels to live against the will of the DNA master does not mean we don't need to have children. In contrast, even when we can live hundreds of years, having and raising children is still one of the most important missions in life. The diversity of the human gene pool is critical not only to the DNA master but also to ourselves. Besides, the DNA master embedded sweet rewards in our genome for creating a new life, which can last for the rest of our lives. Therefore, even as true rebels, our hope for the new generations is still aligned with the DNA master's will. By having children, we fulfill the original meaning of our lives.

Almost all organisms are bothered by aging and death. This deadly problem is almost inevitable since it is written in the genomes and implemented by the embodiments of the DNA master. Therefore, few are competent to do anything about it. In desperate situations, some lifeforms take extreme actions to avoid death. A representative example is cancer cells. Near the end of their normal lifespan, cells sometimes initiate radical remodeling and recombination in their genomes. The DNA molecules are randomly shredded and connected like the making of Frankenstein's monster, which results in highly abnormal chromosomes. Meanwhile, other cellular parts also conduct immense alteration. Most of the transforming cells die in this process while the surviving ones become cancerous and even reach immortality. However, these cells can cause enormous damage to their host, which often leads to tragic endings for both sides. No one wants to take such lunatic actions to extend life since the risk is immeasurably high. Instead, we should gather useful information and create our plan thoughtfully and rationally.

Thus, to become true rebels, our mission is to seek ways to rejuvenate and live healthily beyond the natural human lifespan. We will accomplish this goal systematically with careful learning and sophisticated planning.

Narrow is the way

Many people failed on the way to longer and younger life. Even some of the most powerful and intelligent people didn't reach their goals. However, these forerunners have explored a series of approaches to maximizing the human lifespan and gathered valuable information.

One of the simplest and most common approaches is to have a healthy lifestyle. In practice, many people start with eating healthy food. A modern healthy diet not only means nutritionally balanced but also means organic, grass-fed, no additives, no preservatives, no GMOs, no artificial sugar, no artificial color, no artificial chemicals, no artificial hormones... the list can go on and on. Industrial agriculture has saved human beings from starving, but people turn to foods that are traditionally made for health. Many people believe healthy food reduces unnecessary damage to cells while facilitating proper recovery and maintenance of the body. Although this is at least partially true, healthy food cannot push life beyond its natural limits. No normal person has lived 200 years just by eating and living healthily, except in fairy tales. In China, *Shi Bu* (dietetic invigoration) has been a trendy concept for many thousands of years. One of the core notions of *Shi Bu* is that a person gains what he or she eats. Therefore, the Chinese people eat all kinds of food that they think can revitalize their bodies, some of which are quite bizarre. This concept seems to have developed during ancient times when food was not in abundance. Therefore, the nutritious effects of some edible things were overvalued and no one has yet become superhuman by *Shi Bu*. Nevertheless, healthy food is always popular in different cultures since it is satisfying and relatively easy to obtain. Similarly, healthy lifestyles are also widely accepted. Although healthy lifestyles and foods can improve and sustain a person's health, the benefits he or she gains from them are usually not enough to compensate for what he or she loses through daily life. Thus, the aging process is possibly slowed but far from adequately. For example, the richest and most powerful people can afford the healthiest lifestyle and food. They have specialists to plan their days and experts to cook for them, all guided by professional coaches and nutritionists. However, they do not age much slower or live considerably longer than the rest of the population. It would be fascinating if the natural lifespan boundary could be crossed by eating healthy food and adopting a healthy lifestyle. However, the 3.8 billion years of evolution says no.

A fancier, yet still popular, approach is to get an elixir of life or a magic pill or the holy grail or something similar. Myths from different cultures have described things that can bring health, youth, and eternal life. Many people have a strong belief that such a thing exists in nature. Therefore, for many centuries, people have been looking for such a substance or a few substances to solve the ultimate longevity problem. Interestingly, many of the findings are edible. From the extract of a foreign fruit to vitamin C, the selected substances have been changing but the same idea remains. Just in the past five years, quite a few natural products were claimed to extend the human lifespan and were commercialized. However, some brands did not even last over a year. Evolution does not suggest that such substances exist in nature. Cells and organisms are complex systems with convoluted pathways and mechanisms. The chance that the whole system is dominated by a few substances to produce only beneficial effects is remarkably low. Moreover, footprints of lifeforms have covered almost every corner of this little planet. If some substances can grant organisms superpower or hyper-longevity, their impacts on the evolutionary tree should be obvious. The effects should be at least observable after being accumulated for several billion years. Yet, no evidence has been found so far. Thousands of years of trials and failures indicate that finding the natural elixir of life may not be a winning approach. However, like their precursors, people continue to search for such things, even risking their lives for them.

Although the elixir of life doesn't seem to exist in nature, some people believe that we can develop a wonderful substance through magic, witchcraft, science, or technology. Still, life is elaborate and sophisticated. A simple solution for a complicated problem is an optimistic hope but not always plausible in reality. For example, everyone knows that a single type of food is not enough to provide a full spectrum of nutrients. Thus, people eat all sorts of food, for survival and fun. If the body requires different kinds of nutrients to live each day, it is exceedingly unlikely that a single substance or a few substances can sustain the body and extend life for hundreds of years.

This simple argument doesn't prevent people from attempting to create a magic substance. It could be an enchanted apple, a potion crafted by an alchemist, secret produce from a lost island, an invigorating oil mentioned in an exotic medicine book, or a superfood invented by the most powerful supercomputer that is running state-of-the-art AI algorithms with deep learning and a convoluted neural network plus highly advanced big data analyses. Some people claim that they have used modern technology to develop a single compound which controls a specific enzyme in the body to dramatically increase life expectancy. Even if the target enzyme is the undiscovered silver bullet for hyper-longevity, developing a compound to regulate it accurately and specifically would be very challenging or even impossible. Furthermore, even if the compound can control the target enzyme as claimed, the effects on longevity would be difficult to predict, because the human body is complicated and the variation between people is huge. For example, even the best anticancer drugs are far from 100% efficacy. These medicines are the masterpieces of human biomedical technology. Their development may take 20 years of work by the brightest and most experienced medical professionals. They were tested on thousands of animals and people, costing billions of dollars. They are strictly and continuously regulated and monitored by regulatory agencies from different countries. Despite all the efforts, the effects of many of these drugs still have obvious limitations. Many of them solely target a specific group of the patient population and have expected effects only on a small percentage of patients within the group. At the time this book was written, human beings were engaged in the epic fight with the SARS-CoV-2 coronavirus during the COVID-19 pandemic. In less than a year, the virus infected over 100 million people and killed over 2.5 million victims. Physicians, medical workers, and scientists around the world dedicated themselves to this great work. Yet, the boundary of human medicine was noticeable. The best treatment was the patient's own immune system and the best way to prevent the spread of the virus was implementing lockdowns to block social activities. There was no magic therapy that could instantly eliminate the virus from the patients' bodies. People put their hope in vaccines that were under tortuous development. Likewise, the chance that a magic substance will soon be discovered or developed to extend our lives by 200 years is not promising.

If we cannot expect a magic drug to largely extend lifespan soon, what should we do? Some people think that we should abandon the weakening body once and for all. They have spent millions of dollars on computer science, especially neuron networks and artificial intelligence. The aim is to copy or transfer their mind and memory to reside in a computer hard drive or hard drives (in the cloud). It is a fascinating idea that outshines many sci-fi novels. However, the complexity of the central nervous system is extraordinary. This task won't be any easier than extending the expiration date of the body. Moreover, sufficiently mimicking all the sensory processes and related response networks in a silicon-based system is very challenging. Without senses, a computerized person is no better than carrion locked in a black box. It is hard to believe that this is a superior future to that of an aging body. Without a physical body, inputs from the outside world are simulated by digital signals. However, if it is hacked, the computerized person will be in terrible trouble without knowing it. Instead of a complete transfer, the initial brain computerization could be a simple case of mind copying. Consequently, two or more "copies" of the same person could exist in both the physical and virtual worlds. The relationship between them might be very interesting.

Facing a declining body, some people turn to religious saviors, seeking reincarnation or an afterlife. Similar customs have been practiced since the beginning of human history. This could be a great idea but is beyond the scope of this book. Not trying to be disrespectful, if we just compare the results (if they could be compared), reincarnation seems to have a slice of similarity to transferring the brain to a robot or a cloned body, while the afterlife seems to be somewhat similar to uploading the mind to the cloud. The religious cloud may not have a substantial presence or use up electricity, but an uploaded mind could have a happier and more fulfilled afterlife if the promises are kept. However, the word "afterlife" already reveals the outcome for the body. Nevertheless, faithful people earn miracles like reincarnation or afterlife from their mighty divine saviors.

With so many options, which one should we rely on to extend the existence of our body? I believe the savior of the aging body is the aging body itself. To reach HYL and live 300 or more years, we have to be as one with the only thing that is of us, by us, and for us. By saving the body, the body will save us.

Peeking into the apple

If rejuvenation and longevity were easy to achieve, the world would be filled with 200-year-old "young" people and we wouldn't need to worry about aging and death in our 70s: we could just sit back and relax for another 70 years.

However, even the most powerful people in history have failed to reach HYL, which indicates how difficult it is to find the path. In thermodynamics, energy and power can be easily wasted if the direction of work is unknown. Similarly, even for people who have limitless resources, all the efforts can be in vain if the energy spent is misused. Power with no control can result in nothing, yet knowledge could be the control that gets us to the destination. As illustrated by Maxwell's imaginary demon, knowledge and information can get the work done even in disadvantageous situations. We hope this is still true when we seek a path to HYL.

But where should we start our search? In Genesis, a well-known story describes how humans lost HYL in the first place. Adam, the first man, and his wife Eve took the fruit from the tree of the knowledge of good and evil. Because of this, they were expelled from the garden of Eden. Since the garden was guarded, the couple could not return and eat the fruit of the tree of life. Thus, they lost access to eternity. As a result, they and their descendants, namely all humans, started to suffer from death.

Besides all the significant religious meanings, this is also a magnificent story. I found it insightful and it can help us meditate on the problem we are interested in. What is the meaning of the expulsion? Is it a true punishment or just a test prepared by the owner of the garden? Taking and eating fruits from the tree of the knowledge of good and evil sounds like an unforgivable action. However, expulsion is much gentler than other punishments described in the same book. Neither Adam nor Eve got an immediate death penalty. The punishment Adam received is that he had to work to live, which is quite common for other animals. However, Adam was allowed to live 930 years, an age that any animal would be thrilled to have. The punishment Eve received is that she had increased pain during childbirth. This is very unfair to women, especially given the fact that human babies tend to have large heads. Despite the punishments, the owner of the garden even made clothes for the expelled couple and cared enough to judge the issues of their children. It is hard to believe that this is the attitude someone would have towards people who had committed unpardonable wrongdoing. As constantly expressed in the book, the owner of the garden actually has unconditional love for humans. Given the might of the owner, he could have prevented the expelled couple from coming back to the garden by simply saying so. According to Genesis, his words have absolute power that can even create the world. However, he didn't say anything about it directly. Instead, after sending the couple out, he only assigned guards on the way to the tree of life. Interestingly, there were guards on just one side of the garden. Although the garden was surrounded by rivers, it still didn't seem to be well protected. The security measures might not be adequate for the most important tree in the world. After all, the expelled couple had lived in the garden and should know where they could sneak in without alarming the guards. Moreover, the man had nearly a thousand years to perfect his plan to bypass a security system that was quite crude. Given the great love of the owner of the garden, the expulsion could be a test.

Nevertheless, Adam did not seem to have much zeal for the apples on the tree of life. Rooted in his animal instinct, he should have been afraid of death, especially after seeing the deaths of his kids. However, he demonstrated his compliance for the rest of his life. According to normal human life expectancy, Adam could have suffered at least 200 years of aging and even disability. This is an extremely long period, even on his timescale. It is hard to believe that he did not feel at all desperate about his situation and kindle the desire to put his hands on the tree of life to grab the juicy apples. However, he didn't choose to do a thing. Nor did his wife, kids, grandkids, or any other members of the big family who lived right next to the garden. Adam had almost a millennium to plan for his return, either by tunneling past the guards or secretly crossing one of the rivers. Yet, he didn't even try to talk with the owner of the garden, who might have changed his decision: the owner changed his mind quite a few times in the rest of the book out of his great love of human beings. Moreover, the owner of the garden didn't directly reveal his true intention to Adam, so the real purpose for the expulsion was unknown at that time. It could have been just the opposite of what Adam thought. Even if he was caught during his return to the garden, he could at worst get the death penalty. How could another death penalty be any worse than the one he already had? He had enjoyed exceptionally long years and he had the chance to save his beloved family members, hundreds of them, and his descendants, billions of them. With so many children, even the most timid coward would feel an inevitable sense of duty and find the courage to struggle for their future. However, Adam demonstrates the great virtue of compliance. He buried his curiosity, responsibility, free will, and desire to live even longer. He chose the destiny of a humble servant and earned his longevous life. However, he and his many descendants were thus engraved with the kiss of death and have suffered aging ever since.

Imagine if the expulsion happened in the modern age. Nowadays, there are many ways to gather information about the fruits on a tree in a garden without even getting close to it, at least for normal trees in typical gardens. For example, telescopes, drones, balloons, or satellites can be used to inspect the tree from a distance. It is practicable to illustrate the morphology, color, size, quantity, planting procedure, fruiting cycle, and harvesting method of the tree. These pieces of information can be used to identify similar tree types and prepare for planting once a tree or a seed is obtained. It is possible to find leaves, flowers, seeds, fruits, or even branches of the tree in the rivers near the garden. Modern humans can try to grow the tree, graft the branches for fruits, or clone the plant in their greenhouse. Alternatively, modern humans can chemically synthesize the active ingredient of the fruits, if they can recognize it, or even create something better in flasks through bioengineering. If they cannot obtain specimens from the tree aboveground, modern humans can dig deep underground to track the roots of the tree or analyze soil and water samples. Various technologies can be utilized to investigate the ingredients that compose the tree. The magic substance could potentially be found without directly getting the fruits.

All these imaginary attempts may sound like nonsense. However, isn't this the proper and respectful attitude toward the magnificent tree of life? Aging and death are undoubtedly the most desperate problem for all living beings on Earth. If a physical tree of life could be found, it would be the opportunity to save the lives of *all* humans: adults and children, men and women, of all races and ethnicities, from different countries, cultures, and backgrounds, from now into the future—at least 7 billion in number. Failure means death. Thus, this chance deserves the very best of us to do everything we can to fight for it. At least, that is what the DNA master has been doing for nearly 4 billion years to survive through the cruel insanity of death.

I am not trying or intending to blaspheme or mock religious classics at all. We can make a few tweaks to the brainstorm above so that it is clear how it relates to our topic: the tree of life is the collection of information conveyed by the DNA master; the roots and branches of the tree of life are the essential DNA sequences that support the proliferation and blossoming of lives; the fruit of the tree of life is the essence of all DNA codes, which contains the secret of rejuvenation and hyper-longevity. The fruit is what we have been looking for, which is carried by the species that have been crowned with HYL. They are the leaves, flowers, or seeds of the tree that we found in the rivers near the garden.

Be a copycat

So far, HYL hasn't been achieved by human hands, even with inputs from some of the most powerful and brilliant people. However, some organisms can rejuvenate naturally, live a long life, or even reach immortality. Humans unfortunately are not one of these gifted species, but we can exploit our strength to learn from them and apply it to ourselves.

Quite a few lifeforms have hyper-longevity. One of the best-known examples is turtles, such as the Aldabra giant tortoise (*Aldabrachelys gigantea*). Some turtles can live about 200 years. Therefore, they have become a symbol of longevity and wisdom, and are worshiped in many cultures. Several vertebrates have lifespans that are much longer than those of turtles, including the bowhead whale (*Balaena mysticetus*), Greenland shark (*Somniosus microcephalus*), and others. These species can live from 200 to even 500 years. Invertebrates can live much longer. Some Atlantic seashells (*Arctica islandica*) can live past 500 years while some sponges (*Xestospongia muta*, *Cinachyra Antarctica*, etc.) can live thousands of years.

Some animals, such as *hydra*, appear to be very fragile but have remarkable recoverability and renewability. They don't seem to age or die from aging. Therefore, they theoretically can live a very long time. Lobsters (*Homeridae*) also don't age, though they frequently die for other reasons such as their tastiness. An extreme example of renewability is the immortal jellyfish (*Turritopsis dohrnii*). It repeatedly reverses its biotic cycle to become theoretically immortal. The body of an immortal jellyfish is so frequently replenished that it is difficult to call it

41

rejuvenation since it probably never grows old.

Plants are the true winners of longevity. The longest-living trees (*Pinus longaeva, Taxus baccata, Cupressus sempervirens*, etc.) are even over 5000 years old. However, trees are greatly different from humans: not only in lifestyle, composition, and metabolism but also distinct from us at the cellular level. Invertebrates also share limited similarities with humans. Therefore, though we envy their hyper-longevity, we probably cannot learn as much from them as we can from long-living vertebrates that are closer to us.

Nevertheless, since our goal is to rejuvenate and live 300 years and beyond, who can provide better advice than those who have been through the process and succeeded?

The most important lesson we can learn from these long-living species is that their bodies are capable of living a hyper-long life. This conclusion seems obvious, but it states the fundamental rule of living a hyper-long life: *make sure the body can do it*. If the body by design cannot sustain that many years, there is no way to live that long naturally. The only strategy is to modify the body to make it capable.

This is fundamentally different from the philosophy behind most longevity products on the market. Many dietary supplements, such as the trendy nicotinamide mononucleotide, attempt to maintain the body better so that it can live longer. They may push the body close to or even a little beyond the natural human lifespan. However, even if they work as claimed, the human lifespan won't double or triple. Some people may argue that dietary supplements have successfully extended the human lifespan by a lot in the past 100 years. However, an alternative explanation is that human beings had suffered nutritional deficiency for thousands of years until recently. If the body could not get enough nutrients to build, recover, and sustain itself, it would decay before it should. Therefore, the previously observed human lifespans were much shorter than the actual upper limit determined by the DNA master. With the industrialization of food in the twentieth century, healthy food and dietary supplements now provide enough or extra nutrients to the body so that it can get close to or reach the true natural lifespan. Consequently, it appeared that dietary supplements had dramatically extended the human lifespan. However, it is just the return of human life expectancy to what it should be.

In the current age, nutritional deficiency is no longer a problem for many people. The new generations are filled with all kinds of nutrients, even beyond what they need. Therefore, they should be able to maximize their bodies' natural potential to grow taller, stronger, smarter, and live longer. However, this also means that taking in more nutrients won't boost lifespan much further. Similar cases have been observed in all kinds of domestic and laboratory animals. These animals are well fed and looked after to maintain a healthy lifestyle. They get much better nutrition than their relatives in the wild and are generally much healthier. As expected, they live much longer, even twice or three times more than wild animals. However, they have reached their bodies' natural limits and none of them can extend their lifespans much longer. For example, unless genetically modified, a normal lab mouse can barely live over four years. Even with the popular dietary supplements in their food, mice in longevity experiments cannot live two additional years. Thus, the natural limitation of the body is obvious: a natural mouse cannot live as long as a human, not even close. Some dietary supplements lead to a 10–15% increase in life expectancy for mice tested in studies. If the results can be directly transferred to humans, it means about 7–10 years of increase in human life expectancy. However, these numbers are within the standard deviation of human life expectancy (about 15 years) and the true effects on longevity could be ambiguous. Even if the increase in life expectancy is real, it can be easily ruined by a genetic disorder or a chronic disease. Therefore, such dietary supplements are not capable of extending the human lifespan to our goal.

Both internal (genetic) and external (environmental) factors affect life expectancy. Traditionally, scientists believe genetics contributes to about 25% of the variance in life expectancy, while the majority of the difference is caused by lifestyles. However, if the natural human lifespan is already reached by keeping a healthy lifestyle, the additional beneficial effects of a *healthier* lifestyle become negligible. If a healthy diet and lifestyle could make people live 300 years, many billionaires would have already lived beyond the current human lifespan. As discussed before, such people have enough resources to support the healthiest lifestyle in human history. However, not all of them live beyond 100 years. Interestingly, some of the longest-living people in the world have lifestyles that are quite *unhealthy*. Jeanne Louise, a French woman who lived 122 years, liked smoking, drinking port wine, consuming a lot of olive oils, and eating chocolates throughout her life. Suqing Fu, a woman from China who lived 119 years, ate meat almost daily when she was over 110 years old, especially double-cooked pork (a famous spicy Sichuan cuisine with a lot of fat). Similarly, Yuqiong Wang from China drank alcohol and smoked a lot in her 110s. Although these elderly people may be outliers and the tales may be exaggerated, the stories demonstrate the potential power of the body: certain beneficial genetic variants can overcome the adverse effects of some unhealthy lifestyles. Especially for pushing life beyond its natural limit, some genetic traits and the abilities of the body can become the dominating factors.

Therefore, preparing or modifying the body so that it can live beyond the natural human lifespan is the preferred strategy for hyper-long living. This is conceptually distinct from pushing one's life expectancy close to the body's natural upper limit, which is what most people are trying to do. For reaching our goal, extending the body's capability is a better approach than maximizing its age within its current capability. Just like relocating to a new house, it is much easier to move by getting a big truck than by filling a small car with as many things as possible.

Even for people who only want to live to the natural human lifespan, making the body capable of living much longer is still a preferred strategy. This is due to the potential increase in the marginal benefit of the body. For example, if the body is capable of living 300 years, a 10% increase in life expectancy is 30 years. This is three times the 10% life expectancy increase for a body that is capable of living 100 years. Therefore, extending life expectancy with a 300-year-capable body is more cost-effective than pushing the limit of a 100-year-capable body. To gain 30 years of life, a 100-year-capable body needs to increase life expectancy by 30%, which could be exceedingly difficult to achieve. For the same reason, it is much easier for a human to live one more year than a mouse. Moreover, most humans live greatly longer than the longest-living mouse in the world. Similarly, even if a person with a 300-year-capable body cannot live all the years, it is almost certain that he or she can live much longer than people who are trapped in 100-year-capable bodies. Therefore, it is not reasonable to be penny wise and pound foolish in spending our effort and time, especially when dealing with our own lives.

The prerequisite for living 300 years is to prepare the body so that it can last that long. We have defined HYL as the state that is capable of hyper-long-living. Hence, preparing our bodies to live 300 years is to reach HYL. The question then becomes how to transform the body so that it can live that long, that is, how to achieve HYL.

The long-living organisms are the beacons on the path to

HYL. Our best strategy is to be a humble copycat, following the hints of these thriving precursors. Of course, these organisms are distinct from us. Therefore, we cannot get much lifestyle advice from them and have to use human judgment on this subject. Still, we can identify and follow the common features that are conserved among the many long-living species.

Not surprisingly, none of these organisms achieve HYL with a magic pill or the elixir of life, nor by a healthy dietary supplement or some powerful chemical substances. The answer is already in their DNA when they were born. Modern biotechnologies allow us to peek directly into their genomes and read the secrets written by the DNA master. This is the knowledge that even the great emperors could not get; probably they would have been happy to exchange their enormous power and lands for it.

Despite the dramatic differences between species, these long-living organisms do share a few features. These traits seem to be the cornerstone of their hyper-longevity and rejuvenation ability. For example, many of them have well-maintained telomeres, an effective cancer prevention system, an efficient antidisease network, regeneration at different anatomical levels, vigorous metabolic control, and so on. All of these are recorded in their genomes as gifts from the DNA master. These are the informationized fruits of the tree of life: the secrets of longevity and rejuvenation of 3.8 billion years of evolution, summarized in these model organisms.

We don't get a singular answer to solve our problem: all these model species have multiple features in their bodies to support their long lives. Although everyone likes simplicity, life is complicated. Therefore, it is not surprising that the answer is concise yet systematic. Like Dr. Albert Einstein said, "Everything should be made as simple as possible, but no simpler." What we need is a functional solution rather than a simplistic placebo.

Reaching (and maintaining) HYL implies a hidden mission, which is to decrease the odds of death. This can be achieved by avoiding and managing factors that can lead to death. Reaching HYL and avoiding death are the two sides of the same coin. They can be summarized as two types of procedures: decreasing AELH and increasing AELD, respectively (Figure 6). Accordingly, the lessons we have learned from the long-living organisms are divided into these two categories. Thus, ten tasks (five for each category) are described as *the roadmap to HYL* (Figure 6). These tasks are listed from simple daily items to more difficult and complicated assignments. Tasks in these two lists need to be accomplished simultaneously.

I. To reach HYL by decreasing AELH:
A. **Healthy lifestyle** to balance metabolism and properly maintain the body.
B. **Telomere maintenance** to ensure the health and longevity of cells.
C. **Tissue regeneration** to replenish cells, tissues, organs, and organ systems.
D. **Neural maintenance** to improve the health of neurons and nervous systems.
E. **Systematic coordination** to precisely adjust different cells, tissues, organs, and organ systems to keep them healthy and functioning properly for a long time.

II. To avoid death by increasing AELD:
1. **Danger prevention** to stay safe and avoid risk factors to reduce the chance of sudden death and damage to the body.
2. **Routine genome maintenance** to eliminate DNA lesions to diminish problems caused by damaged DNA and unhealthy cells.
3. **Treatment of diseases and disorders** to minimize damage and manage risks for cells, tissues, organs, and the body.

4. **Tumor suppression** to eliminate cancerous cells.

5. **Systematic coordination** to ease genetic risk factors and suppress issues of different body parts.

Figure 6.
The roadmap to HYL.

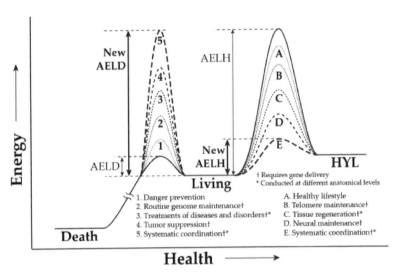

The strategy to reach HYL consists of a series of tasks. These tasks either decrease AELH (tasks A–E) to make HYL more accessible or increase AELD (tasks 1–5) to reduce the odds of death. The goal is to reach HYL and maintain the self-stabilizing balance in HYL to live beyond the natural boundary.

The roadmap illustrates a systematic approach to adapting the human body to a hyper-long life that is beyond its natural limit while maintaining its optimal condition (Figure 6). The goal is to reach HYL, a self-stabilizing balance that is constantly replenished. In this state, the body has enhanced recoverability, renewability, and regenerability with enlarged lechatelierim. HYL is reached by repeated rejuvenation and renewal of the body. First at the cellular level (task B), then for tissues and organs (tasks C and D), and finally replenishing the whole body (task E). Meanwhile, a risk detection and suppression network is established at different anatomical levels of the body (tasks 2–5). It is used to constantly monitor, identify, manage, and eliminate potential risks to the body. By avoiding death and sustaining health, the body is kept in HYL and thus capable of prolonged living. Last but not least, maintaining a healthy lifestyle (task A) and avoiding environmental risk factors (task 1) facilitate survival beyond the natural human lifespan (Figure 6).

As a general guide for rejuvenation and longevity, this roadmap has its limitations. To simplify the roadmap, it starts from a normal living state. Therefore, potential inherited genetic disorders and other diseases are not considered as initial conditions. Moreover, rejuvenation is prioritized in the roadmap, which may not apply to some people. For example, youngsters and people with some genetic traits don't need to get young again, though they still need to maintain their status. Besides, the roadmap is designed according to current knowledge of life sciences and biotechnologies. Although the tasks seem fundamental, people may find a distinct route to reach HYL and live 300 or more years. In the future, biotechnology could be so developed that people are customized to perfection when they are still a zygote. Many of these customizations are probably related to the tasks in the roadmap. At that time, all our current worries will be superfluous and the roadmap no longer necessary.

Does the roadmap guarantee rejuvenation and a life that is longer than usual? Of course not. As discussed earlier, the probability of a reaction is crucial but out of our control. By decreasing AELH and increasing AELD, we reduce the odds of death and maximize the likelihood of reaching HYL (Figure

6). However, it is possible that things eventually don't work out and a person fails on his or her path to HYL. Moreover, almost all reactions are reversible. If a person reaches HYL, he or she could still exit that state and even enter death. Repeated or continuous maintenance of the body may help to prevent this from happening, but the huge energy gap between life and death still makes the natural process unidirectional and spontaneous (Figure 4). Even for a person who has been in HYL for a very long time, death will eventually bring him or her to eternal serenity.

Therefore, should we trust the roadmap? I believe so. It is derived from the organisms that have successfully reached HYL and lived hyper-long lives. These are the best models we can find on Earth in the past 3.8 billion years. Hence, we should be able to trust the roadmap, at least more than some other approaches. However, should we follow the roadmap? I don't know. But if you choose to, that will be a lifelong journey.

The Diamond Drill

Mei you jin gang zuan, jiu bie lan ci qi huo.
(Don't take china works if you don't have the diamond drill. /
Don't work on a project if you don't have the appropriate
tool.)
—Chinese proverb

By copying the strategies of the DNA master's masterpieces, the
roadmap to HYL illustrates a path to our dream. However, can
it be accomplished with current human technology? Or do we
still need to wait for a diamond drill?

What the world needs most

The two lists in the roadmap contain tasks with ascending
difficulties. The easiest ones are to look out for danger and
maintain a healthy lifestyle, while the most challenging ones
require performing precise and systematic adjustments of
different body parts at will. Current technology cannot fully
accomplish all the tasks in the roadmap. However, even partially
fulfilling some tasks is beneficial for longevity. For example,
telomere maintenance has rejuvenation effects on the cells and
can largely extend the theoretical life expectancy. Partially
accomplishing these tasks will buy us time to wait for science
and technology developments that lead to the completion of the
roadmap.

What is the fundamental technology for the roadmap?
Many of the tasks require precise manipulation of genes and
coordination of cellular processes using DNA. As demonstrated
by the DNA master, these actions need the expression, inhibition,
modification, and adjustment of specific DNA fragments. Since
we are copying the masterpieces of the DNA master, we should
conduct similar works like *It*. Therefore, we need to send a lot of

commands to cells. These commands are coded in DNA or RNA (ribonucleic acid) fragments. Hence, a gene delivery system that is capable of efficiently and reliably delivering specific nucleic acids into human cells (through transfection or transduction) is at the core of the roadmap.

This technology is the essential diamond drill as described in the Chinese proverb at the beginning of this chapter: without it, we cannot complete the roadmap to reach HYL.

Since a gene delivery system can also send genes to treat diseases, it may sound similar to gene therapy. However, it is quite distinct from current gene therapy. And thus, gene *delivery* is used to emphasize the differences.

First, gene delivery is not just for therapies. Treating diseases and disorders is just a small part of its numerous applications. In the roadmap, many tasks are routine checkups or maintenance. Rather than treating diseases and disorders, these applications are more like conditioning one's hair or conducting skincare. In the future, a fully developed gene delivery system could be so easily accessible that it is used daily for all kinds of trivial things. Therefore, the hypothetical applications of gene delivery are much broader than the current definition of gene therapy. Second, gene therapy usually targets an organ or a specific body part. However, gene delivery is not restricted to limited areas of the body or certain cell types. To accomplish some tasks in the roadmap, the messages encoded in DNA or other nucleic acids need to be sent to most, if not all, cells in the body. Moreover, systematic coordination requires the delivery and regulation of a wide variety of genes. These concepts are beyond the scope of current gene therapy. Last but not least, to complete the roadmap, different DNA or RNA molecules need to be frequently and repeatedly sent to cells. This is difficult to achieve by current gene therapy strategies. Hence, gene delivery in the roadmap is distinct from traditional gene therapy.

A fully developed gene delivery system will bring enormous changes to our daily life. The functions of many drugs are performed through stimulating specific cell receptors, which affect certain cellular pathways to coordinate the expression or inhibition of some genes. If we can deliver the same gene or its inhibitory piece to cells, it should induce similar effects to those of the corresponding drug. Drug development is conducted case by case for individual receptors, which can take 20 years to mature and may not succeed after all the efforts. In contrast, designing functional DNA or RNA to express or inhibit genes is a mature technology and can be readily applied to new targets. Coding DNA or RNA fragments is also much easier and less costly than designing, screening, developing, and synthesizing a drug. Therefore, we could have various specific DNA or RNA pieces to cover all kinds of health issues. Similarly, DNA or RNA vaccines can be designed and prepared faster than traditional vaccines. For example, in the COVID-19 pandemic, the first vaccines used in the USA were messenger RNA (mRNA) vaccines. Moreover, a fully developed gene delivery system can be widely used in our daily life. For example, we can use it to adjust our metabolism to work more efficiently or improve the quality of life.

With such a gene delivery system, we can regulate our genes almost freely. Therefore, I believe it will be the world's best technology ever. We will use it as the diamond drill to treat the world's deadliest disease: aging.

En route

If a gene delivery system that is suitable for the roadmap is so powerful, when will we have it? It probably won't take too long, but it won't be too quick either. Chances are we will see it soon in our lifetime.

Scientists and engineers have developed various gene delivery systems. There are mainly four types, categorized by transfection methods: physical, chemical, viral, and naked nucleic acids. Some technologies also utilize a mixed methodology. Physical methods use physical forces to temporally open holes in the cell membrane to facilitate cargo (nucleic acids of interest) delivery. This can be achieved through a tiny sharp needle (microinjection), high voltage electrical field (electroporation), the bombardment of high-speed particles (gene guns), and other methods. Chemical methods utilize a broad variety of reagents such as inorganic compounds, liposomes, nanoparticles, and so on. These reagents form particles or complexes with the cargo, protecting the nucleic acids from degradation. The particles or complexes then adhere to the cell surface or merge into the cell membrane, releasing the cargo into the cell. Viruses can naturally introduce viral genetic materials to host cells. By incorporating the cargo into the viral genome, the engineered virus becomes a carrier to deliver the cargo into the target cells. Naked nucleic acids such as normal or chemically modified DNA and RNA can also be directly injected into tissues for transfection. Many of these gene delivery technologies have been commercialized and are in widespread use.

However, these transfection technologies still have inevitable weaknesses. Some technologies are very efficient on cultured cells, but cannot easily be applied to the human body. For cultured cells, transfection efficiency is the most important factor; this is what drove the early development of gene delivery technologies. However, additional factors have to be taken into account for *in vivo* applications such as delivering nucleic acids in live animals. Safety becomes the primary concern and restricts the application of many technologies to higher organisms such as human beings. The major safety factors of transfection technologies include toxicity, compatibility with the cell growth environment, side effects on cell structures and functions, immunogenicity, biodegradability, and so on. Technologies with safety concerns cannot easily be used on the human body, though many of them are highly effective.

Using the transient poration mechanism, physical methods can achieve desirable transfection efficiency. However, these methods may trigger cell death and require complicated instruments. Thus, *in vivo* applications are limited. For example, electroporation causes severe cell damage and leads to extensive cell death. If it is used on the human body, it requires the insertion of high voltage electrodes into the tissues. Therefore, its usage is likely to be limited.

Many chemical transfection methods are very effective in cultured cells. However, their efficacy is hindered by the complicated *in vivo* environment, especially due to the nonspecific interactions of serum and other proteins. Moreover, many chemicals, polymers, and nanoparticles used for gene delivery are toxic. Consequently, they raise major safety concerns when being applied to people, especially for reagents that cannot be degraded by the human body. Besides, some toxic lipid-based chemicals can become incorporated into the cell membrane and be trapped for a long time. Thus, their applications have potential health concerns.

Certain viruses have great gene delivery efficiency in the human body, such as retroviruses, adenoviruses, adeno-associated viruses (AAVs), lentiviruses, and others. Hence, they have been used for various gene therapies. Since these viruses only recognize and deliver to certain cell types, most virus-based gene therapies target a defined body part. A major disadvantage of viruses is immunogenicity. These viruses can be relatively easily identified and neutralized by the immune system. Consequently, it is likely that they can only be used once, or not at all, during a person's lifetime. Viruses naturally have the potential to infect the host and cause adverse effects. Besides, viruses can quite frequently incorporate viral genes into the host genomes, which then last for a lifetime. Viruses also have cargo constraints and only deliver DNA or RNA fragments that are smaller than a certain size. Moreover, these engineered viruses are also expensive and complicated to make, which further limits their applications.

Naked nucleic acids have low immunogenicity and toxicity. However, they also have low transfection efficiency and a high degradation rate. In recent years, several gene therapies using modified RNA have been approved. However, they are very short fragments and can only be used for inhibiting specific genes. The manufacture of these RNA fragments is very pricey and the treatment can cost over half a million dollars per year.

Due to the many issues of current gene delivery technologies, they have limited applications on the human body. Thus, gene therapies are mostly chosen by desperate patients with life-threatening diseases. They are also used under emergency use authorizations for public health crises. However, the utilization of gene delivery on healthy human beings for nontherapeutic applications, such as in some tasks of the roadmap, should follow the highest safety standards ever set.

The delivered DNA or RNA is degraded not long after gene delivery. However, current gene delivery technologies cannot safely support continuous or frequently repeated transfections to the human body. Therefore, if a long-term genetic change is required, the delivered gene needs to be incorporated into the genome of the target cell. There are several methodologies to conduct genetic modification, but most of them are complicated to operate. The simple CRISPR-Cas systems are thus popularly used in gene therapies. However, these systems have frequent off-target effects, which lead to the modification of a random region of the genome instead of the target region. Dangerous consequences can result if the modified region encodes a critical function. Since the off-target rate is up to 50% and there are 37 trillion cells in the human body, conducting genetic modification on the whole body is likely to result in serious problems using current technologies.

Therefore, quite a lot of development is still required to obtain a desired gene delivery system and related technologies that we can use to complete the roadmap to HYL.

Just one step at a time

Although our current technologies cannot fulfill the requirements needed for the roadmap, gene delivery systems will probably be sufficiently advanced soon to support the pursuit of youth and longevity. Before such a technology is developed, we can frame the essential features of an ideal gene delivery system. This also highlights the problems of current methods, which have to be solved before they can be widely used on healthy human beings.

Since the gene delivery system will be used on people, safety is the top priority. It cannot have detectable short-term or long-term toxicity to the human body at the amount used. Even at the extreme dosage used to transfect all the cells in the body, it needs to be well tolerated by the person to enable repeated usage. It also cannot have obvious cell toxicity to the cells that are transfected. Besides cell death, other cytopathic effects should also be avoided, such as damages to cell structure, disruption of cell function, prevention of cell growth, and so on. If it is a chemical-based gene delivery system, the reagents used would preferably be biodegradable. Thus, if the chemicals were left in the body, the unpredicted effects can be minimized.

Besides safety concerns, an ideal gene delivery system should be compatible with the *in vivo* cell growth environment so that it is suitable for the human body. The reagents or devices used should fit the human body without causing pain or other uncomfortable feelings or problems. The gene delivery system needs to deliver a large number of nucleic acids to the whole body without disrupting metabolism. A methodology also needs to be developed so that the transfection can cover the whole body. At the cellular level, the gene delivery system cannot disrupt cell metabolism and proliferation. Therefore, the transfection condition used should be mild and avoid disrupting the internal and external environments of cells.

An ideal gene delivery system also has to be efficient *in vivo*. The human body is complicated and filled with all kinds of biomolecules. Serum and other proteins reduce the efficiency of many current transfection technologies. An ideal gene delivery system should have a well-designed transfection mechanism to ensure its effectiveness in interfering environments. Moreover, the transfection process needs to be completed as quickly as possible.

Low immunogenicity is another essential feature of an ideal gene delivery system. Once recognized by the immune system, the resulting immune response can be dangerous and severely impede the transfection process. Moreover, the immune system is likely to prevent all future transfections. Consequently, repeated gene delivery, which is required for the roadmap, is hindered. Therefore, an ideal gene delivery system has to have low immunogenicity.

An ideal gene delivery system should not be restricted by cargo size. Larger DNA and RNA pieces can load more useful information to the cell, which is important for completing tasks in the roadmap. Therefore, an ideal gene delivery system should be able to deliver nucleic acids of a large size. Besides, the gene delivery system should not introduce unnecessary foreign genes to the target cells. Foreign DNA can be intentionally or unexpectedly incorporated into the human genome during the transfection process. This not only contaminates the human gene pool but also puts the host in unknown danger. Foreign DNA incorporation can cause serious problems when many cells are transfected at the same time and lead to disastrous consequences.

The transfection protocol should be as simple as possible. If the procedure is complicated, the failure rate and the risk of problems will greatly increase. It is also easier to evaluate the results of a simple process. Moreover, a simple protocol may also reduce the time required to complete the procedure.

An ideal gene delivery system should also be versatile for future engineering. According to the roadmap, systematic coordination needs precise adjustments of different cell types. Each cell type may require additional upgrades of the gene delivery system to increase transfection specificity and efficacy. Therefore, a system that is convenient for further engineering can easily cater to a variety of needs and tasks. Moreover, high engineering versatility also facilitates further development and improvement of the system.

The manufacture of the gene delivery system should also be as simple as possible. Repeated whole-body gene delivery will require huge amounts of reagents and consumables. A simple manufacturing procedure enables timely large-scale production. It also reduces the materials and manpower required, leading to more reliable manufacturing and simplified quality control. Thus, it may dramatically reduce the manufacturing cost.

These are the essential features of an ideal gene delivery system that is capable of accomplishing the tasks in the roadmap. For simplicity, such a gene delivery system will be referred to as a Miao ("wonderful" or "clever" in Chinese) system in the following chapters. A perfect Miao system can be hard to develop. Fortunately, the tasks in the roadmap have different complexities. Many of the tasks do not require a complete Miao system. Therefore, a developing or primitive Miao system can be used to accomplish the simple tasks in the roadmap. The person can then wait for a more advanced Miao system with his or her extended life expectancy. Nevertheless, even a prototype Miao system needs to satisfy the majority of the essential features, especially safety.

The development of a Miao system can have several stages to

fulfill different requirements. A hypothetical development plan is described as the following.

Level 0: A safe and efficient Miao system that is sufficient for use in cultured cells. Such a Miao system can be used for some gene therapies and immunotherapies.

Level 1: A safe and efficient Miao system that is sufficient for use in certain cells or specific parts of the human body. Such a Miao system can appropriately target and transfect certain cell types in the human body.

Level 2: A safe and efficient Miao system that is sufficient for use on the whole body to transfect all or most cells. Such a Miao system can appropriately target and transfect all the major cell types. However, its usage on a few specific cell types could still be limited.

Level 3: A safe and efficient Miao system that is sufficient for use on the whole body to precisely target specific cells. Such a Miao system can appropriately identify, target, and transfect the desired cell type or types, specifically and precisely.

A level 3 Miao system is ideal for accomplishing all the tasks in the roadmap and maintaining HYL for a long time. It is the diamond drill we are looking for.

All set to go

A safe, reliable, and efficient gene delivery system is our ticket to HYL. However, we have to wait for a suitable Miao system to become available. It could come soon, or it could take 20 years, though not likely. Hopefully, it will be developed before it is too late for us.

While waiting for technology advancement, it is important to know what needs to be done to reach HYL. The details of the tasks in the roadmap are explained in the following chapters, through which we can become familiar with what to do once the technology is developed. Meanwhile, we can work on the simple tasks in the roadmap to maintain and improve our bodies. Based on science and technology developments in the past 20 years, the waiting won't take long. Let's be prepared and get ready to work our way to healthy youthful longevity.

Scientia potentia est.

II. Xing
(Actions)

The roadmap illustrates a path to HYL. Now let's discuss how to deal with the tasks in the roadmap with a suitable Miao system.

Table 1.
Chapters in Xing and tasks in the roadmap included in each chapter

Chapter	AELH task	AELD task
The Tail-chasing Telomere	B	
Cancer Catcher		2 and 4
Recover, Renew, and Regenerate	C	
Diseases and Disorders		3
The Enemies from Outside		3
Forward to Basics	A	1
Neuron, A New Frontier	D	
The Ultimate Balance	E	5

The Tail-chasing Telomere

Lost time is never found again.
—Benjamin Franklin

All lifeforms have embodiments of the DNA master inside their cells. These DNA molecules form the genomes of different organisms. There are mainly two types of DNA: circular and linear (Figure 7). The human genome is the linear type.

Do you hear the tick-tock sound?

The biggest difference between the two types of DNA is that the linear DNA has two ends (Figure 7). This makes it less stable and more vulnerable to hydrolysis or degradation. During DNA replication, the two ends of linear DNA are not fully covered by DNA polymerases for synthesis. Thus, the two ends are trimmed each time the cell divides. The shortening in human cells is up to 300 bp per cell division and the loss accumulates over time. If genes with important functions are deleted during this process, the cell could be in huge trouble. Therefore, evolution creates telomeres.

Telomeres are the regions at the two ends of linear chromosomal DNA (Figure 7). There are repeated DNA sequences that do not contain any protein-encoding gene. In human beings, the repeating sequence is 5'-TTAGGG-3' and each telomere contains about 2,500 repeats (15,000 bp). The primary function of telomeres is to label and protect the ends of the chromosomes. The telomeres are marked and distinguished from other DNA ends in chromosomes, such as double strand breaks that need repair. Therefore, the DNA repair proteins won't accidentally link the chromosomal ends together to create a giant Möbius loop. Instead of losing genes with important functions, some redundant telomeric repeats are deleted each time the DNA replicates. The DNA master thus found a quite sloppy solution for this eukaryotic cells' life-or-death problem. Nevertheless, the essential parts of the genome are protected as long as the telomere is still long enough to withstand the replication lost. When a cell replicates enough times to reach the Hayflick limit, its telomere is too short for more cell division. Consequently, further replication is ceased and the cell enters the state of senescence. In this state, the cell moves towards its final destination: it can self-destruct by programmed cell death, or send inflammatory signals to attract immune cells to terminate it. In some respects, the telomere is like a roll of toilet paper. People use it periodically to deal with messy troubles but no one worries about it until the paper is running low. Eventually, when all the paper is used up and the empty roll is exposed, the problem becomes serious and the panic escalates.

Figure 7.
Circular and linear DNA.

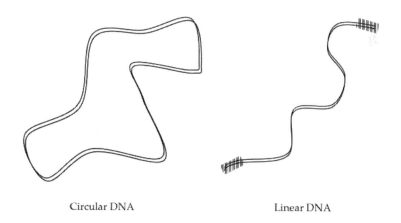

Circular DNA   Linear DNA

The shadowed regions at the two ends of the linear DNA are its telomeres.

A telomere is protected and sensed by various types of

proteins. By checking the telomere length, they monitor the health status of the cell and determine how many replications the cell can still live through. A cell ages as telomeres shorten after each cell cycle. An aged cell, like an aged human, starts to have more problems. Its protein expression pattern and metabolism differ, while waste and DNA damage accumulate. Gradually, the recoverability of the cell loses to the chaotic trend of molecules and the balance inside the cell becomes unstable. Hence, it has an increased possibility of surpassing AELD and starting the death procedure. The cell senses the survival pressure and it needs to react or it will die eventually. The only opportunity is to become cancerous. Similar to humans and other lifeforms, some cells take the path of a rebel to fight against destiny, while some just give up and die.

To struggle for survival, cells with short telomeres initiate a harsh transformation, including a series of desperate actions. Some cells turn off tumor suppressor proteins and activate alternative cellular pathways to extend their lives. Some cells continue to replicate even without a telomere and trim off functional genes. Some cells fuse the different chromosomal DNA ends to generate messy chimeric DNA. These abnormal DNA molecules are then randomly divided during replication, causing serious mutations and damages. Many cells die during this process. Few cells elongate their telomeres to bypass the Hayflick limit and finally reach theoretical immortality. They become cancerous and, if the environment allows, can duplicate indefinitely. One of the most famous cancer cells is the HeLa cells, which have been preserved in laboratories around the world since 1951, the year when their host passed away because of them.

If we were created by some supreme beings, the existence of telomeres probably indicates that they don't want us to live forever. This could be because they love us so much that they would like us to return to them after a definite time. The relation between telomere length and estimated lifespan has been confirmed by a series of studies. It is consistent in most eukaryotes such as animals and plants. The telomere is just one of the many dedicated molecular clocks that the DNA master created. To us, the shortening of telomeres is like a countdown to death, since a person cannot keep living if cells in his or her body are aging and dying. Every year, the telomeres in the human body drop about 70 bp on average. Cold but consistent, this reminds us of the time that has flown by. Some scientists refer to the human leukocyte telomere length of 5,000 bp as the telomeric brink, since people with telomeres shorter than that have a great risk of imminent death.

Telomeres provide a natural cap on everyone's life. However, people are *not* born equally. Some people are born with longer telomeres; thus they get a longer theoretical lifespan as a gift at birth. Some people, unfortunately, are born with shorter telomeres; thus they face a potential loss of 10 or 20 years of life at the beginning. The difference in telomere lengths contributes to the variance of human life expectancy, which has a standard deviation of about 15 years. Currently, there are commercial products available to measure a person's telomere length to estimate the number of years he or she has left.

For humans, the maximum lifespan predicted by telomere length is about 100, plus a few years. Based on the shortening speed of the human telomere, people with the ability to live 300 years need nearly 2 million bp of telomeres in all chromosomes in a cell. This is about 0.07% of the 3 billion bp human genome, which is not a small percentage for a repeating sequence. In ancient China, emperors were honored with the title *Wan Sui*, which means "living to 10,000 years." Life this long requires a total telomere length of about 64 million bp in a single cell. Given that the average length of a nucleotide is about 0.6 nanometers and the human body has 37 trillion cells, the total telomere length of *Wan Sui* could reach 1,430,000,000,000 meters

(888,560,804.90 miles). This is about the distance between Saturn and the sun.

Just hope we can turn back time

If the shortening telomeres correlate with aging, cancer, and death, why not make them longer? The DNA master probably had the same thought. Fortunately, evolution created a sophisticated machine to extend telomeres, which is the enzyme named telomerase.

The function of telomerase is very simple. The enzyme adds the same repeats to the end of telomeres to grow them. Once telomeres are elongated, the number of divisions the cell can conduct increases. This means the aging process of the cell is reversed. Thus, the cell rejuvenates and no longer has urgent survival pressure. Theoretically, cells can become immortal with sufficiently active telomerases. This sounds like the silver bullet against aging and death.

Telomerase is a highly conserved protein that can be found in almost all eukaryotes with linear chromosomal DNA. It is in plants and animals, as well as humans. However, cells in our bodies still age and die. This is because telomerase is highly regulated in normal cells and cannot be activated freely. In most cells, telomerase is barely expressed or not expressed at all. Thus, only a small number of active enzymes exist so that telomere elongation is highly restricted. In contrast, many cancer cells have lots of active telomerases, which enable them to duplicate indefinitely and live forever. Since active telomerases are more abundant in cancer cells than normal cells, they have been used as targets to recognize cancer cells. Various drugs and therapies have thus been developed to precisely kill cancer cells by recognizing telomerase.

Although telomerase is common in cancer cells, active telomerase does not turn cells cancerous. In contrast, it may decrease the chance of carcinogenesis. Since active telomerase reduces the survival pressure of cells, stress response pathways that can lead to tumorigenesis are not stimulated. Many long-living animals, like the bowhead whale and Greenland shark, maintain functional telomerases in cells. These active enzymes enable the healthy duplication of their cells for several hundred years and facilitate tumor suppression during that long period. Unfortunately, we the people are not one of the few species that continuously express telomerase. If we were made by some supreme beings, for this reason, I would be sad about being disfavored and would envy the long-living animals. Nevertheless, active telomerase is the central prerequisite for rejuvenation and longevity. It is a must-have on our path to HYL.

If telomerase is so important, can we manually activate it? Dr. María A. Blasco at the Spanish National Cancer Research Center has conducted a series of investigations into telomerase and aging. Her group has shown that lifespan in different species can be predicted by the telomere shortening rate. They also demonstrated the beneficial effects of telomerase against aging.

The study most relevant to the roadmap is her research on activated telomerase. In this work, she conducted AAV-based gene therapy to activate telomerase in mice. The adult and old mice that received gene therapy had an increase in lifespan of about 24% and 13%, respectively. These percentage changes are about twice the standard deviation of human life expectancies in corresponding age groups. These numbers are also much higher than the results of most dietary supplement longevity studies. If the outcomes can be repeated in humans, it means 10–30 years of extra life. An even more exciting result is that telomerase gene therapy does not promote tumorigenesis, which has been tested for various cancer types in multiple follow-up studies.

Dr. Blasco also studied the effects of hyper-long telomeres on longevity. Mice born with hyper-long telomeres have a lifespan increase of about 13% and reduced cancer incidence.

Although the increase is still impressive, mice born with hyper-long telomeres have less gain in lifespan than adult mice that received telomerase gene therapy. These results have indicated that active telomerase may be more effective than existing long telomeres in extending lifespan. Accordingly, with active telomerase, people born with short telomeres may have a longer lifespan than people born with long telomeres. These studies have also demonstrated that extra life acquired by technology, such as through telomerase gene therapy, can overcome innate boundaries predetermined by nature to obtain advantages. Thus, these results support the strategy of using telomerase gene therapy to extend the theoretical lifespan.

In Dr. Blasco's experiments, the mice only received one injection of telomerase gene therapy. Since the transfection efficiency in normal mouse gene therapies was only 20–50%, a single injection is a long way from covering most mouse cells. Even with this obvious caveat, a remarkable lifespan expansion was achieved. It is reasonable to believe that repeated administrations of telomerase gene therapy to cover most or all cells will result in an even bigger boost in lifespan. However, due to immunogenicity, the same AAV injection can only be utilized once. Therefore, a Miao system that can be repeatedly used is required to maximize the power of telomerase gene therapy. Moreover, the effects of gene therapy wear off over time due to the degradation of the delivered gene. Genetic modification or recurrent administration may thus be needed to maintain the activation effects to increase lifespan further. Hence, a Miao system will be essential for prolonged or repeated activation of telomerase.

The collected works of Dr. Blasco have demonstrated the importance of telomerase in longevity and established the key role of telomerase gene therapy in increasing lifespan. Gene therapies to elongate telomeres have already been applied to the human body. BioViva, a Washington-based biotechnology company, conducted AAV-based telomerase gene therapy on its CEO, Elizabeth Parrish. However, the result is ambiguous: the extended length of her telomeres is still within the variation of the measurements. Gene therapy is certainly more difficult in humans than in mice. Since the human body is greatly bigger than a mouse body, a single injection covers a much smaller percentage of cells in humans. Even though the transfection efficiency of AAV-based gene therapy in humans is similar to that in mice, it is more challenging to cover most cells in the human body. Therefore, even if the telomere elongation effect on Elizabeth Parrish is real, it is likely that only a tiny percentage of cells in her body have received the benefits. Unfortunately, she doesn't have a second chance to have the same therapy.

Therefore, it is probably not a brilliant idea to take AAV-based telomerase gene therapy soon. The major concern is that the same AAV can likely be used only once in a person's life. If the once-in-a-lifetime treatment failed or had ambiguous results, regret would be the only thing left. It doesn't seem to be worth the risk until the telomerase activation technology is fully developed. Ideally, the technology will mature before long and everyone will get the chance to extend their lives. If a person took the shot too early and lost the only chance, he or she would then watch others live happily ever after in great sorrow. Moreover, the same AAV can also be used for gene therapies against cancer or other serious diseases. It does not seem to be the correct choice to waste a life-saving opportunity on matters that are not urgent yet. Not until a better gene delivery system is developed.

Nevertheless, in 2019, Libella Gene Therapeutics launched a clinical trial for AAV-based telomerase gene therapy in Colombia. This is a patient-paid trial and the cost of the therapy is 1 million USD per patient. It could be worth it for people who want to take the chance.

Keys of the kingdom

Active telomerase is fundamental for reaching HYL. The activation of telomerase in our bodies is the ticket to start the journey. Listed as task B in the roadmap (Figure 6), it is the cornerstone of living beyond the natural boundary.

Current AAV-based gene therapy has its limitations. Issues such as high cost and complicated manufacturing procedure can be overlooked; the risk of incorporating viral genes into the human genome can also be mostly ignored. However, immunogenicity is the Achilles' heel of AAV and most other viral transfection systems. This inevitable problem restricts the usage of the same gene therapy: it can be used only once, if it can be done at all.

However, a single injection is unlikely to transfect all or most replicating cells in the human body. A human is about 2,000 times heavier than a mouse. Thus, according to weight-based dosing, AAV required for humans needs to be 2,000 times the amount used on mice. Calculating based on mice studies, this requires about 4 quadrillion (10 to the power of 15) viral genomes of AAV. AAV transduction efficiency is generally 20–50%. If only 20% of a person's body can live 200 years while the rest cannot, it is unlikely that he or she can live that long. Therefore, to compensate for insufficient transduction efficiency, the injected amount has to be doubled or even decupled to cover most cells in the body. The required AAV is thus 8 to 40 quadrillion viral genomes. Such a huge amount of AAV can weigh 0.25 grams (the average molecular weight of AAV is 3,746 kDa). Since the typical concentration range for AAV gene therapy is 0.01–0.1 mg/mL, the injection volume can range from 2.5 to 25 Liters. Even if everything could be packed into a single injection, the syringe size would be very scary. Even by intravenous infusion, it might take weeks to administer all the AAV. Given that the average volume of the human body is about 65 Liters, it would be challenging to evenly distribute all the injectants in the body in a timely fashion. However, with a Miao system that is capable of repeated administration, gene delivery could be conducted multiple times until most cells have active telomerase.

Recurring telomerase activation will be required for a 300-year lifespan. According to Dr. Blasco's mice studies, telomerase activation has about twice the effect in increasing lifespan than hyper-long telomeres, which is still far from doubling the mouse lifespan. Therefore, even if hyper-long telomeres are generated by a single gene delivery treatment, it is unlikely to increase lifespan by several hundred years. Thus, repeated telomerase gene delivery is likely to be the only practical way to push the theoretical lifespan over 300 years.

Figure 8.

A tentative plan for extending theoretical lifespan to 300 years by repeated telomerase gene delivery treatments.

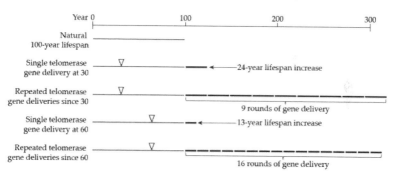

According to results in mice, for a person with a 100-year natural lifespan (thin lines), a single telomerase gene delivery can increase his or her life by 24 or 13 years (thick lines) if administered at the age of 30 or 60 (triangles), respectively. Thus, this person needs 9 or 16 rounds of repeated telomerase gene deliveries to extend his or her lifespan to 300 years.

If Dr. Blasco's mice studies can be repeated in humans, a single injection of telomerase gene therapy can lead to a human lifespan increase of about 24%. This means 24 extra years of life for people with a 100-year natural lifespan (Figure 8). Although a 124-year lifespan is remarkable, it is not even close to 300 years. If the extended telomere length is comparable in each telomerase activation treatment, it is reasonable to assume that the lifespan increase is also similar after each gene delivery treatment. Thus, to achieve a 300-year lifespan, a person with a 100-year lifespan needs at least 9 rounds of whole-body telomerase gene delivery treatment (Figure 8). This is greatly beyond the capability of current AAV-based gene therapies.

Another interesting finding in Dr. Blasco's mice studies is that a greater lifespan increase is obtained if the telomerase gene therapy is conducted at an earlier age. Old mice that received telomerase gene therapy only had a lifespan increase that was barely half of that in adult mice. This result could be due to the aging of the mouse body or the nature of the gene therapy. Assuming the results are repeatable in humans, it means a person with a 100-year natural lifespan has only a 13-year lifespan increase if he or she receives telomerase gene therapy in his or her 60s. This increase is 11 years less than the increase he or she can have if he or she receives the same therapy in his or her 30s. Consequently, to achieve a 300-year lifespan, a person needs at least 16 rounds of whole-body telomerase gene delivery if he or she starts in his or her 60s (Figure 8). The number of rounds he or she needs then is about twice the number needed if he or she starts in his or her 30s. The increased cost and treatment complexity resulting from more rounds of gene delivery could be a problem. Besides, more risk factors appear when a person gets older, which creates more uncertainties for the treatments. Hypothetically, if the body is greatly rejuvenated after the first treatment, the following treatments may provide larger lifespan increments. Thus, fewer than 9 rounds of treatment may be enough to achieve a 300-year theoretical lifespan regardless of starting age. However, it is unclear if the treatments of a rejuvenated body will lead to larger lifespan increments. It is also difficult to predict the best age to start receiving telomerase gene delivery that maximizes lifespan increase. The optimal age may vary among individual people.

Thus, a dilemma about waiting for technological advancement occurs. The older a person gets, the more developed gene delivery technology he or she can expect. However, the lifespan increase he or she can get from a single (at least the first) telomerase gene delivery drops. This dilemma may be solved by repeated or recurrent gene delivery using a Miao system.

Developing a suitable gene delivery system is not the only challenge for having active telomerases in our cells. Even if the transfection is adequate, issues with the delivered gene can still prevent successful gene therapy. Telomerase is highly regulated, which means this enzyme requires the coordination of a series of cofactors to support folding and functions. Therefore, simply forcing cells to express telomerase may not get functional enzymes. Moreover, telomerase can be rapidly degraded if it is not in active use. Thus, even if the functional proteins are present in cells, their degradation could be so rapid that they cannot catalyze any reaction. Elizabeth Parrish's ambiguous gene therapy result could be due to any of these reasons. The only way to know the exact cause is through detailed molecular analyses to dissect the mechanism of telomerase.

This is not a simple science question. Discovered by Dr. Carol W. Greider and Dr. Elizabeth Blackburn in 1984, telomerase has been extensively studied by multiple Nobel laureates and many other world-class researchers. After more than 35 years, human telomerase remains one of the most difficult enzymes to work with. Its unstable nature leads to rapid precipitation and degradation. Thus, human telomerase still has difficulties being expressed and purified in large quantities for research and drug screening. Therefore, detailed structural and mechanistic information on human telomerase remains to be determined. To complete task B in the roadmap, scientists probably need to design and engineer an active telomerase that is less regulated by its cofactors.

With a suitable telomerase and a sufficient Miao system, we should be able to periodically extend our telomeres. Thus, the aging process of our cells will be reversed and we will rejuvenate from the cellular level. According to Dr. Blasco's mice studies, we will also get fewer cases of damage in our DNA, have better metabolism and a reduced chance for cancer, and live longer. Even with an incomplete Miao system, a successful gene delivery system is likely to provide 20 years of extra life. Given the current speed of technological development, this is quite a long time for the advancement of a potential Miao system. At that point, it will provide a better gene delivery experience for the second and subsequent times. Eventually, we will periodically repeat the telomerase gene delivery treatment until our goal is reached many, many years later.

Cancer Catcher

Failure is not an option.
—Gene Kranz, at Apollo 13 mission control

Cancer is always one of the leading causes of death. It takes millions of lives every year. Chances are, if a person lives long enough, he or she will get cancer eventually. Thus, dealing with cancer is a major task in both normal life and HYL.

The game of stochasticity

When cells become abnormal, they can grow and divide uncontrollably. As a result, cancer starts. (Details that distinguish cancer and tumor are beyond our scope of discussion. Therefore, the terms "cancer" and "tumor," including benign tumors, are used interchangeably for simplicity.) This abnormality is caused by DNA mutations.

DNA is a stable molecule with an extremely long half-life. However, the information it carries can be easily manipulated. This simplifies the recording, modification, and copying of the book of life, but is prone to mutations. From the DNA master's perspective, mutations are good. The diversity of life is created by mutagenesis. It helps organisms to climb out of the prebiotic soup and conquer the entire Earth. Millions of distinct species have been evolved by mutagenesis to adapt to different environments, for the continuation of the DNA master and for their own survival. However, for an individual organism, mutagenesis can also be bad. It carries the hidden curse that one's own body will turn against itself and result in death.

Figure 9.
Carcinogenesis and countermeasures.

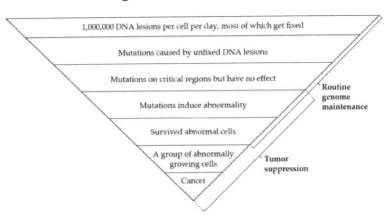

In the human body, there are about a million DNA lesions per cell per day (top). Most of them get fixed or have trivial effects. However, some of them become critical mutations. The accumulation of these mutations could make cells grow abnormally and develop cancer (bottom). In the roadmap, two tasks focus on different steps of this process to sense abnormality and eliminate cancerous cells.

Numerous things can cause DNA damage and lead to mutations, which can be categorized into external and internal factors. External factors include ultraviolet from the sun, X-rays and other radiation, toxic and mutagenic chemicals, certain viruses, and so on. Internally, byproducts from intracellular metabolic pathways, such as reactive oxygen species (ROS), can damage DNA. Consequently, the DNA nucleotides can be deleted, mutated, modified, mismatched, crosslinked, or formed into weird conformations. More seriously, one or both strands of DNA can be broken, crosslinked, or trapped in complicated structures. Besides, instances of DNA damage are spontaneously introduced in natural cellular pathways such as DNA replication and DNA recombination. During these processes, errors can be incorporated into the genome, DNA strands can be broken, and different DNA fragments can be mixed up randomly.

Therefore, DNA damage occurs very frequently. It is estimated that each human cell has about one million DNA lesions per day (Figure 9). Given that we have about 37 trillion cells in our bodies, on each day the body gets 37,000,000,000,000,000,000,000 new instances of DNA damage. This is an astonishingly large number. If we assume lesions are always distributed on different residues, then about 0.02% of our 6-billion-nucleotide genome is damaged daily. Based on this assumption, all residues in our genome will be damaged or mutated within 17 years.

Fortunately, most DNA damage gets fixed. To protect the vulnerable embodiments of the DNA master, cells evolved a comprehensive network of DNA repair proteins not long after abiogenesis. From bacteria to human beings, a highly conserved system guards the integrity of the genome every day. There are multiple DNA repair pathways, each targeting specific types of DNA lesions. For example, base excision repair corrects damaged single bases and nucleotides, homologous recombination repairs DNA double-strand breaks with homologous overhangs, non-homologous end joining fixes DNA double-strand breaks with blunt ends, and so on. A large number of proteins are involved in these repair pathways. Some proteins participate in a single pathway, while some are shared among different processes. Moreover, each repair pathway contains multiple steps to repair a DNA lesion following strict protocols. For example, DNA mismatch repair is the main pathway to correct DNA replication errors, which reduces replication lesions by 1,000-fold. This is a three-step process that has been illustrated by Nobel laureate Dr. Paul L. Modrich and other distinguished researchers. First, a group of proteins recognizes the DNA lesion and attracts other proteins. Then, the arriving proteins remove a DNA fragment containing the DNA lesion. Finally, a different group of proteins resynthesizes the DNA fragment with the correct DNA sequence. As a result, the accurate coordination between different proteins fixes the DNA lesion.

The collected efforts of different DNA repair proteins safeguard the integrity and stability of our genome. These dedicated workers protect our cells and our lives. However, just too many cases of DNA damage are generated (Figure 9). If a person lived 100 years, he or she would have about 1,350,500,000,000,000,000,000, 000 DNA lesions throughout his or her life. This number is over a million times larger than the population of all insects on Earth. Even our sophisticated DNA repair pathways cannot cover all of them and unfixed DNA damage stochastically occurs. The DNA repair system also makes mistakes and can introduce errors into the genome. Moreover, when the body gets older, the efficiency of the DNA repair system decreases. Consequently, the incidence rate of unfixed DNA lesions increases.

Most unfixed or wrongly fixed DNA damage leads to mutations (Figure 9). Thus, information recorded in the genome is modified. Fortunately, a major part of the genome is not that important. The mutations may not occur on genes or regions that have critical functions. Even if a mutation lands on an important region, it may not create any change or the change is trivial. Even if the change is significant, it may still be within the lechatelierim of the cell and causes no problem (Figure 9). However, even with so many "even"s, one random mutation can land on a critical position of an essential gene, which introduces abnormality to the cell. This happens randomly: it may occur when someone is 18 as the first mutation in a critical cell of an important organ, or it may occur as the nine-billionth mutation in an insignificant cell in someone's 90s. A single mutation can start the carcinogenic process, but the probability is low. Usually, the accumulation of many mutations gradually drives the abnormal transformation until the process is irreversible

(Figure 9). Hence, the possibility of getting cancer increases over time. When people live long enough, cancer seems inevitable.

Even when a cell becomes abnormal due to the accumulation of dangerous mutations, things are still under control. The cellular network of DNA damage response not only senses DNA damage to induce DNA repair but also contains various signal pathways. These signal pathways respond to DNA abnormalities, especially during the cell division cycle. Through the cell cycle, there are multiple checkpoints. At each checkpoint, DNA integrity is assessed by checking a series of requirements by a group of regulatory proteins. If a cell fails to pass the assessment, it cannot proceed to the next phase of the cell cycle to complete cell division. Therefore, damaged or incomplete DNA won't be transferred to daughter cells. If DNA abnormalities cannot be resolved, DNA damage response pathways can initiate suicide procedures such as programmed cell death or attracting immune cells to destroy the cell. Consequently, the abnormality is terminated by the death of a single cell without causing bigger problems for the body.

However, if critical genes of the DNA damage response or related pathways are mutated, things become complicated. In this case, the abnormal cell cannot get exterminated but instead continues to replicate itself. The more it duplicates, the higher the chance of introducing additional mutations to the genome. Consequently, the abnormal cell can become cancerous and pass the abnormality to more daughter cells. This chain reaction may end up in a benign tumor that is almost completely harmless to the body. Alternatively, it may become invasive and result in life-threatening cancer (Figure 9).

In this game of stochasticity, no one knows for how long he or she can remain as a lucky winner until the deadly bullet arrives unpredictably.

Backups of backups

After years of development in cancer biology and therapies, cancer remains one of the most lethal human killers. Several cancer types can be cured with great success rates, even prevented by vaccines. However, the deadliest cancer types are still dangerous and nearly impossible to treat. A few cancer types have a less than 1% five-year survival rate. If these cancers are in the terminal stage, patients can hardly survive for longer than three months. In these extreme cases, it is difficult to plan for a 300-year life.

Therefore, the best strategy is to avoid cancer as much as possible and eliminate it when it is still trivial. This mission has to be a top priority for long life in HYL. Thus, two tasks in the roadmap (Figure 6) exist for this purpose: routine genome maintenance (task 2) and tumor suppression (task 4).

Routine genome maintenance

The critical role of DNA repair in maintaining genome integrity for health and longevity has been demonstrated in many studies. Species with long lifespans tend to have more effective DNA repair systems. However, the enhancement varies among species and a universal approach cannot be identified. Some species have more copies of DNA repair genes, some species have elevated DNA repair gene expression levels, some species have more frequent DNA repair checkups, and some species have more efficient DNA repair proteins. To achieve HYL, genome integrity needs to be maintained for a long time. A simple strategy is to increase the efficiency of our DNA repair system following the pattern of these long-living animals.

One approach is to increase the copy number of DNA repair genes, as seen in bowhead whales. It is expected that more gene copies generate more active enzymes. However, there are so many DNA repair proteins and supporting proteins to facilitate different pathways. Even with a perfect Miao

84

system, it is challenging to increase the copy numbers of all the proteins in all cells in the body. Therefore, at least at the beginning, only a limited number of genes should be selected for this approach. The selection can be based on the frequency and severity of types of DNA damage. The most common types of DNA damage are DNA replication errors, ROS damage, depurination, and single-strand breaks. These types of damage occur over a thousand times per cell per day. Double-strand breaks occur at a much lower frequency but can bring serious damage to the cell. However, just those types of DNA damage listed above are repaired by over 20 different proteins from five repair pathways. Therefore, the selection for gene delivery won't be easy. Once the proteins of interest are selected, their genes need to be delivered to all or most cells in the body. Thus, at least a level 2 Miao system is required for this task. Similar to telomerase activation, repeated or recurrent gene delivery is needed to ensure most cells are transfected. After gene delivery, some cells may have more gene copies than others, which can lead to gene expression variation between cells. It is unclear if any adverse effect can be induced by too many copies of DNA repair genes. However, keeping gene copy numbers the same or similar in all cells seems reasonable. There are ways to limit gene copy numbers in cells, but detailed planning is needed before conducting gene delivery. Since DNA repair pathways are frequently catalyzed, the additional gene copies need to be kept in cells for a long time. This can be achieved by incorporating the delivered copies into the genome by genetic modification or keeping them as extrachromosomal DNA, each of which requires sophisticated design.

Another approach is to directly elevate DNA repair gene expression levels, as seen in naked mole-rats (*Heterocephalus glaber*). These animals are the longest-living rodents and can live 10 to 15 times longer than normal mice and rats. Increasing gene expression levels can be achieved by two different methods. One method is to modify or switch the gene promoter. A promoter is the DNA sequence that initiates and regulates the expression of a gene. An improved promoter can raise gene expression levels. The other method is to deliver regulatory proteins or substances that can boost gene expression by interacting with the specific promoter. Either method can be achieved through gene delivery. Genetic modification of specific promoters may be required in this process. By using gene delivery, elevating gene expression levels faces similar challenges as increasing gene copies. Since many proteins function together in DNA repair pathways, the expression levels of all of them need to be adjusted collaboratively. It may lead to an unbalanced increase in expression levels if the adjustment is not even. This may cause unpredicted issues such as precipitation of proteins or alteration of DNA repair pathways.

Inducing more frequent DNA repair checkups is another approach to improve DNA repair efficacy. This can be achieved by modifying specific genes in the regulatory pathways. Similar to the other approaches, it may require genetic modifications to incorporate the changes into the genome.

We can also introduce more efficient DNA repair proteins into our cells. Some animal DNA repair proteins contain mutations to make them more effective than corresponding human proteins. These genes are positively selected in evolution and can usually be found in long-living animals, such as some sharks. These species need reliable DNA repair systems to prevent carcinogenesis for several hundred years. Therefore, replacing our genes with homologs from these animals is likely to boost our DNA repair efficiency. However, these exogenous genes probably need further engineering to make them adaptive to human cells.

As the first line of defense, routine genome maintenance reduces the DNA mutation rate and helps our cells live healthily for a long time with a decreased chance of carcinogenesis (Figure 9).

Tumor suppression

With a long lifespan, even the most efficient DNA repair system cannot prevent DNA mutations from accumulating and cells from developing cancerous abnormality. Despite its rareness, cancer has been found in at least 20 kinds of sharks. Therefore, identifying and terminating cancerous cells is crucial for HYL.

Most cells utilize a network of tumor suppressors, cell cycle proteins, and other regulatory proteins to sense DNA mutations that are the direct cause of carcinogenesis. If a cell becomes abnormal, these pathways can shut down cell proliferation and conduct suicide. By monitoring DNA abnormality, these pathways can detect threats at the early stage, and eliminate potential dangers even before cancer cells develop. This critical mechanism also works in cancer cells. Thus, activating or re-activating these pathways is a promising strategy to treat and cure cancer. If these natural anticancer pathways can be routinely activated, they will become an effective cancer prevention and suppression mechanism.

Such a mechanism can be established with a suitable Miao system. The main strategy is to activate more tumor suppressors, cell cycle proteins, and other regulatory proteins. Similar to routine genome maintenance, this can be achieved by delivering more gene copies, increasing gene expression levels, inducing more DNA checkups, or using more effective proteins.

For example, a straightforward approach is to periodically deliver tumor suppressor p53, which is encoded in the TP53 gene. Famous for being "the guardian of the genome," p53 has excellent anticancer effects. It actives DNA repair proteins to fix DNA lesions and halts the cell cycle if DNA damage is not corrected or when the telomeres are short. Moreover, it initiates programmed cell death when DNA damage cannot be reversed. Since p53 is so powerful, its malfunction has devastating consequences. Mutations of the TP53 gene occur in almost every cancer type. Thus, gene therapy to replace mutated p53 with functional p53 is one of the first anticancer gene therapies. Moreover, multiple drugs have been developed to target mutated p53, aiming to reactivate its function or recognize cancer cells.

If losing p53 is so terrifying, a simple solution is to have multiple copies of the TP53 gene. This is exactly what elephants have; it is their secret. African elephants (*Loxodonta africana*) have 20 more copies of the TP53 gene than humans. Therefore, the p53-induced programmed cell death (apoptosis) is much more frequent in elephants than humans to remove abnormal cells. With a similar lifespan to ours, elephants rarely get cancer and their cancer-caused death rate is also much lower (< 5%). Therefore, it is reasonable to believe that p53 gene delivery can greatly enhance tumor suppression effects in our bodies. Similar to routine genome maintenance, possible approaches are to incorporate more copies of the TP53 gene into our genome, elevate its expression level, or introduce more effective homologs. Since only one gene is involved, tumor suppression using p53 gene delivery is much simpler.

The development of cancer from abnormal cells is much slower than the occurrence of DNA lesions. The process can take weeks or even years. Thus, constant activation of the TP53 gene by genetic modification or extrachromosomal DNA may not be necessary. Monthly, quarterly, or even annual p53 gene delivery may be enough to eliminate abnormal cells from the body. Such procedures are like periodical computer antivirus scans. A level 2 Miao system should be adequate for this approach to suppress carcinogenesis. With routine p53 checkups, cancer is unlikely to occur. Even if it develops, p53 gene delivery can be used to eliminate it.

A suitable Miao system can also be used for different kinds of cancer therapies against various cancer stages. A level 0 Miao system can be used for immunotherapy. A level 1 or level 2 Miao system can be used to conduct targeted therapy or hormone therapy. A level 1 or higher Miao system can aid known cancer therapies such as surgery, radiation therapy, chemotherapy, and stem cell transplant by delivering proteins to facilitate recovery or suppress side effects. It can also be developed into novel anticancer therapies by activating tumor suppressor genes, inhibiting overexpressed cancer genes, correcting cancer mutations, guiding immune cells to attack cancer cells, or commanding cancer cells to eliminate themselves. However, with all the risks associated with cancer, prevention is still the best cure.

Nevertheless, to reach and maintain HYL, multiple lines of defense should be established to prevent and fight cancer.

The principle of the DNA master

Cancer cells are our cells. Thus, it is challenging to distinguish them from normal cells but it is easy for them to spread in the body. This feature greatly increases the difficulty of cancer treatment.

The recognition of cancer cells can rely on their external traits such as abnormal morphology, secretions, or receptors on the cell surface. However, these external features are diverse among cancer cells and the recognition specificity varies. Thus, immunotherapies that train immune cells to accurately recognize and eliminate cancer cells have become trendy. However, the results differ between cancer types and therapeutic strategies.

Some cancer therapies recognize cancer cells using their internal metabolic changes. For example, cancer cells proliferate much faster than most normal cells. Thus, many chemotherapies target DNA replication proteins to eliminate rapidly dividing cancer cells. However, this also imperils other replicating cells, such as hair cells and hematopoietic stem cells (blood-forming cells) in the bone marrow. Therefore, hair loss and anemia are the common side effects of these chemotherapies. Some cancers are induced by the malfunction of important tumor suppressor or DNA repair genes. Thus, drugs and specialized therapeutic strategies based on these mutations have been developed. Some breast cancer subtypes are well-known examples, which have achieved great therapeutic success.

The variation between cancer patients can be huge. Cancers originate from DNA mutations, which are stochastically distributed over the 6 billion residues in the human genome. This creates exceptional randomness and causes differences between patients. Moreover, the diversity of the human body and metabolism further enlarges cancer variation. Consequently, it is common for patients to obtain different results from the same treatment. Since a single strategy is unlikely to succeed in all patients, personalized medicine has become the future of cancer treatment. Supported by the rapid development of gene-sequencing technologies, personalized medicine develops detailed therapeutic strategies based on a patient's specific mutation types.

The principal difference between cancer cells and normal cells is in their DNA. However, the cell is still the only one that can check its genome for abnormality and react accordingly. Its pathways are the most accurate diagnostic devices and the most effective anticancer tools. Therefore, we should utilize tumor suppressor pathways in cancer cells to fight against themselves. Many therapeutic strategies and drugs have been developed to activate tumor suppression pathways. With the help of a suitable Miao system, we can increase the power of such pathways to identify and eliminate cancer cells.

When we kill cancer cells, we are killing a part of ourselves. We do this for the benefit of the majority, the one who runs the brain, which we believe is the "true" ourselves. Thus, by doing this, we have quietly accepted the doctrine that the rights of the many outweigh the rights of the few. Strictly speaking, we don't even care about the needs of the few in the case of cancer cells. This is remarkably similar to the principle of the DNA master: individuals are dispensable for *Its* existence and evolvement.

Cruel as it may sound, we eliminate cells we no longer need throughout our life. It makes us who we are. For example, the development of the nervous system and fingers is accomplished by removing *lots* of cells from the crude prototypes. Otherwise, we could not feel and touch this world. In the circle of life, decomposed bodies of dead organisms are recycled and resurrected in the bodies of new lives. Similarly, in our bodies, biomolecules from dead cells are reused in new cells. However, unlike us, the mindless DNA master cannot designate the death of a particular organism or species.

It is tangled yet interesting that we are using the principle from which we would like to escape in order to escape from the same principle. Sadly, this is the secret of survival that the DNA master has learned from 3.8 billion years of struggling. The organisms and species that survived the extinctions are the ones who sacrificed their lives for their lives. Many lifeforms have faced tradeoffs and learned the important lesson that they have to pay the cost of one thing by giving up something else. For example, some trapped animals even chew off their own feet to escape with their lives. In some respects, dealing with cancer is something similar. No matter whether DNA lesions will become mutations or not, they have to be corrected. No matter whether cells with abnormality will become cancerous or not, they have to be eliminated. Not taking any risks is the only way to survive this game.

Recover, Renew, and Regenerate

That is no country for old men.
—William Butler Yeats, 'Sailing to Byzantium'

All things wear out. An aged body is no longer a young body. Dealing with this spontaneous process is an ongoing task on our way to reach and maintain HYL.

Mind the mileage

As deadly as it is, cancer is not the No. 1 cause of death. Cardiovascular diseases have been the worldwide winner in taking human lives. Killing almost twice as many people as cancer, they have been keeping the first place for over 30 years. Many cardiovascular diseases are due to the accumulation of waste and the wear on the cardiovascular system after years of use. Similarly, many other diseases that are leading causes of death are also initiated by the erosion of the corresponding systems over a person's lifetime, such as some respiratory diseases, liver diseases, kidney diseases, and digestive diseases.

In some respects, the human body is like a car. Both things are essential for our daily life and accompany us for many years. To keep up the performance of a car and ensure the safety of people in the car, routine maintenance is essential. Periodically, oil and filter need to be changed, and tires and brakes need to be adjusted. After a long time, a more thorough service is required. Worn wires, belts, tires, glass, fluids, and other parts need to be replaced, while clogs, stains, and short circuits have to be removed. Otherwise, my old Camry that broke down in the middle of an interstate highway could be the result.

In the service years of the old Camry, the solution to most of its problems was quite simple: replacing the worn parts with new ones. Its tires, battery, wipers, headlights, transmission fluids, and stereos were not the original ones. They were replaced and worked well, just like in a brand new car. The old Camry got extended life with these new gadgets. Sadly, the shimmering "check engine" light had been unintentionally ignored. Later, the old Camry's engine began to scream with loud clacking and popping noises one day on the highway. Even after that, the old Camry could still have been saved if the engine had been replaced. Our bodies are unfortunately not as well maintained as my old Camry. The old car received many services and replacements, but we cannot do similar things to the body.

Like a car manufacture warranty, the human body has a network of systems to inspect and repair potential malfunctions. For example, cells are continuously renewed by a series of cellular pathways. The organs use metabolism to exchange biological materials with the outside world to maintain a healthy state. The body can recover from small wounds and injuries within its lechatelierim. However, for a car, even a bumper-to-bumper warranty doesn't cover all types of damage. If the damage is too severe, insurance companies need to be called. Similarly, the body cannot recover by itself from serious injuries and illnesses. If the problem is close to or beyond its limit, we need to see a doctor. Hence, we should follow LeChatelierism and minimize damage to our bodies. Besides, issues accumulate over time. For either a car or a body, an aged one gets more problems. After the expiration of the manufacturer's warranty, more services are required but the performance continuously drops.

Many cardiovascular diseases are caused this way. After years of use and wear, the blood vessels become thinner. They are more fragile and lose elasticity. Clogs gradually develop from years of accumulation of fats and plaques, which is the Sword of Damocles hanging over the circulatory system. Consequently, coronary and peripheral artery diseases and stroke may be induced. Similarly, years of endless pumping of the heart can lead to congestive heart failure, arrhythmia, or cardiac arrest.

When people get old, other organs face the same problem: slower metabolism reduces recoverability and renewability while the accumulation of waste hinders normal functionality. For example, our lungs are like two large air filters. However, far from replacing them twice a year like the ones in a car, we cannot even clean them easily. Decades of smoke, dirt, chemicals, pollens, mucus, and things that were accidentally sucked in are all trapped inside the lungs. The lung cells cannot tolerate these foreign objects but cannot get rid of them either. Thus, immune responses are triggered, scars are formed, alveoli die, air exchange function gradually drops, and chronic obstructive pulmonary disease develops. The liver and kidneys have similar issues.

Nowadays, many drugs target specific receptors to prevent the propagation of diseases or to relieve the symptoms. However, the reversal of the disease process is still almost impossible. Similarly, stenting or coronary artery bypass surgery eases the symptoms or creates alternative solutions, but the damaged or clogged tissue cannot be renewed. Several new technologies, which are still under preliminary development, claim to clean clogged blood vessels.

The best solution so far is to replace the damaged tissue or organ. The new one can be taken from another part of the body or from a donor, or be in the form of an artificial organ or regenerated biomaterials.

Replacement from another part of the body is rarely possible for critical organs. Thus, transplantation from a donor is a common and practical approach. However, not all organs can be transplanted, while finding an appropriate donor is always difficult. For many transplantations, donors need to have matching tissue types and other biological markers. Therefore, waiting for an appropriate donor can take many years. Transplant surgery is also challenging. Even if the surgery is successful, transplant rejection, graft-versus-host disease, and other side effects are common issues that could be lethal. Nevertheless, transplantation still saves and extends patients' lives, so tens of thousands of people are eagerly waiting for donated organs.

Therefore, xenotransplantation, which is transplanting tissues or organs from another species, has been developed to fill the shortage of human donors. Although cells from other species are likely to induce severe immune responses, genetic modifications of donor animals are supposed to relieve such effects. Artificial organs can be another substitute for donated organs, as well as tissues and organs produced from regenerated biomaterials. However, the development of these technologies is still in the preliminary stage, and extensive improvement is still required to precisely replicate the natural functions created by the DNA master.

Regenerated tissues or organs can be made from stem cells. These are cells with the ability to develop into other cell types. The most potent stem cells are embryonic stem cells from embryos, which are difficult to obtain and have possible ethical issues associated with their use. Scientists have developed induced pluripotent stem cells from adult cells that have partial functions of embryonic stem cells. However, regenerating tissues or organs with stem cells remains a challenging research question. For example, organ printing is a relatively new technique to generate tissues or organs by putting different types of cells together, but this is still not developed enough for real transplantation.

Due to the supply shortage, transplantation is still mainly limited to patients with serious diseases. For healthy people who pursue HYL or want to replace a used but not damaged organ, it would be difficult to find a donor. Meanwhile, due to the many potential side effects, the benefits of the surgery don't seem to outweigh the risks, at least for now.

Used (like new)

Even in HYL, the wearing down of the body after living a long time is an unavoidable problem since the body itself cannot recover from all the damage accumulated over the years. This problem can be both microscopic and macroscopic, but neither can be easily solved by simply delivering a few genes. If a healthy lifestyle is maintained, we don't need to worry too much about this problem for a long time. However, plaques or clogs in blood vessels and wastes trapped in organs will have to be physically removed someday during a 300-year or longer life. Otherwise, transplantation would be required eventually. As task C in the roadmap (Figure 6), the recovery, renewal, and regeneration of the body needs to be conducted at multiple anatomical levels.

At the cellular level, genome integrity should be maintained at a healthy level by recurrent gene delivery of DNA repair genes as described in previous chapters. Elongated telomeres and activated signal pathways can reverse the aging of cells and keep them in a "young" state. Consequently, cells can effectively reduce the amount of molecular wastes accumulated inside them through enhanced metabolism and recover from damage caused by chemical oxidation.

The activated cells can continuously renew themselves while properly conducting cellular functions, which could help to recover, renew, and regenerate the nearby tissues. Gene delivery of specific growth factors can further induce cell proliferation to aid tissue healing. It is unclear if rejuvenated cells can induce regeneration at the organ level. Many functional cells have differentiated into specialized cell types for their functions. Consequently, they no longer divide or proliferate. Thus, keeping differentiated cells healthy and functional alone may not reverse the existing damage and wear in the organ.

In some organs, cell proliferation is conducted by stem cells. Somatic stem cells are stem cells found in different parts of our bodies, which can proliferate and differentiate into multiple cell types of a special lineage. Embryonic stem cells are much more powerful and can theoretically differentiate into all cell types in the body. The challenges of utilizing stem cells after harvesting include proliferating them to the required amount and guiding them to differentiate into desired cell types. A level 0 Miao system can facilitate the culture of stem cells outside the body. In combination with other reagents, repeated gene delivery with different signals should be able to induce the proliferation and differentiation of stem cells. However, there exist several challenges in practice. For example, the timing of gene delivery is complicated. The expression of delivered genes can take hours or even days, which may not align with the cell cycle of stem cells. Moreover, the coordination between various external reagents and gene delivery of multiple genes is not simple. Systematic screening and testing are required for optimizing conditions to proliferate and differentiate cells.

Even if various cells can be cultivated in large amounts, developing a functional organ is more challenging. Nevertheless, creating a complete and functional organ directly from a small pile of stem cells in a Petri dish would be the ultimate solution for organ regeneration. However, gluing different cells together cannot generate a real organ that can live and have functions. Making a working organ in a test tube probably requires the precise replication of the *in vivo* organ development processes by simultaneously consolidating the growth of multiple cell types. It needs a comprehensive understanding of the development and mechanisms of different cells in an organ. It also requires the sophisticated distribution of intracellular and intercellular signals, while maintaining a growth environment similar to the human body. Thus, a level 3 Miao system that can accurately deliver genes to specific cell types would be essential for completing this challenging mission. Once a functional tissue or organ is synthesized *ex vivo*, transplantation can still be risky. Furthermore, the transplant has to live and function properly inside the body. Therefore, an alternative strategy is to directly grow a new organ inside the body by stimulating stem cells to proliferate and differentiate. However, the coordination of multiple gene deliveries *in vivo* would be more complicated. Moreover, the safety precautions are more complicated, yet there is no room for risk or failure.

If we cannot turn cells into organs, xenotransplantation will be the most feasible solution for the near future. Although the donor shortage may be solved, the massive difference between species remains the biggest problem. Some researchers have been using genetic modifications to make model animals more "human," aiming to reduce transplant rejection and side effects. An appropriate Miao system surely can facilitate this process. However, even if all animal genes related to an organ are replaced with the corresponding human genes, the animal organ is still unlikely to be the same as the human organ. The organ that grows inside an animal is constantly affected and altered by the animal's *in vivo* environment to ensure the survival of the animal. Hence, to develop a human organ inside an animal, the related organ systems may also need to be humanized. This can be as challenging as guiding the direction of evolution. Still, it is difficult to determine how "human" the donor animal should be to provide usable organs for xenotransplantation.

Alternatively, maybe a technically simpler approach is to make humanoid donors, probably developed from genetically modified human embryos. In an ideal world, these humanoids would have an exact human *in vivo* environment to grow functional human organs, but, to make such a deed ethical, they cannot have consciousness, intelligence, senses, feelings, or even a brain. However, the brain and senses are likely to be essential for the humanoid's development and thus cannot be eliminated. Consequently, no matter how life-saving it could be, the debate and criticism surrounding such an approach will be furious. The principal problem would be: How "nonhuman" must a humanoid be to avoid ethical blame, while being "human" enough to serve as a valid organ donor? However, a proposal to experimentally study such a question will be immediately banned by even the most open-minded ethical committee in the world.

Although difficult, organ regeneration may not be a great concern in HYL for a long time. After all, all the beings who have lived to 300 years on this planet have relied only on the recoverability and renewability of their cells. None of them even know about transplantation.

Diseases and Disorders

Medicine heals doubts as well as diseases.
—Karl Marx

Everyone gets sick sometimes in life and it is inevitable in the long years of HYL. Thus, dealing with diseases and disorders is task 3 in the roadmap (Figure 6). The World Health Organization (WHO) has published the *International Classification of Diseases*, which records about 55,000 unique codes for injuries, diseases, and other causes of death. Some disorders and diseases are reviewed in other chapters and to cover all of them is beyond our scope. In this chapter, we will discuss the general strategies for handling some of the conditions.

Ailments

With elongated telomeres, proper DNA maintenance, regenerating cells, and active organs, a person in HYL should have a larger lechatelierim than average people. However, greater recoverability doesn't prevent him or her from getting sick. Luckily, modern medications have protected people from most ailments. Even over-the-counter medicines can take care of most daily problems.

If a Miao system is developed enough to greatly lower its cost, it will have the potential to replace or compensate for many common drugs. For example, ibuprofen is a common nonsteroidal anti-inflammatory drug used for pain relief and fever reduction. The main function of ibuprofen is to inhibit two enzymes: COX-1 and COX-2, which are the key enzymes in prostaglandin biosynthesis. COX-1 is constantly expressed in cells, while COX-2 is expressed during inflammation. Ibuprofen inhibits COX-1 and COX-2 to block multiple pathways that use the products of these two enzymes. Gene delivery can be used

100

to inhibit the expression of these two enzymes or subsequent enzymes. The inhibition can be accomplished by many approaches, such as using antisense oligonucleotides (ASOs) to block protein synthesis or expressing mutated proteins to compete with normal enzymes. Such inhibition should have comparable effects to those of ibuprofen.

Similar approaches can be used for many other medicines. For example, over 30 different antihistamines target histamine H_1 receptors, such as loratadine, cetirizine, diphenhydramine, fexofenadine, and others. They are all commercialized and can be found in most drugstores. The receptor coordinates several intracellular signaling pathways. Inhibiting proteins on these pathways by gene delivery can suppress specific pathways to obtain a similar effect to these antihistamines. Moreover, the delivered gene could be maintained in cells to provide more sustained effects than rapidly excreted small-molecule drugs.

The effects of gene delivery are likely to be slower than drugs. Thus, it may not be suitable for relieving acute conditions but for alleviating symptoms over a longer period. For example, local growth factor gene delivery can facilitate and accelerate the healing of serious wounds such as diabetic foot ulcers. Similar gene therapies have been tested in several clinical trials.

Chronic conditions

Repeated or recurrent gene delivery and genetic modifications are potential solutions for many chronic conditions.

One example is chronic pain. Local gene delivery to inhibit nociceptors (pain receptors) can suppress unbearable pain. In extreme cases, these receptors can even be permanently shut off by incorporating modifications into the genome. A level 3 Miao system would be preferred for such treatments, but even a level 1 Miao system could be used if it is applied to a defined region of the body. These therapies should be able to eliminate the most severe feelings of pain. More excitingly, it wouldn't cause addiction, poisoning, or other adverse effects, all of which can be provoked by the commonly used opioids.

Another example is Type I diabetes. Patients with this condition have an impaired pancreas and can no longer produce enough insulin. Consequently, they have to periodically inject insulin into themselves for the rest of their lives through pens, syringes, or pumps. The frequent injections can be both uncomfortable and tedious. However, it could be life-threatening if the periodical injections are interrupted. Gene delivery or genetic modifications can be used to command patients' cells to secrete insulin. The cells do not need to be in the pancreas since many cells are capable of synthesizing peptidyl hormones if the appropriate genes are delivered. The muscle cells on the butt or arms may be good choices, but the secretion amount requires careful adjustments. The patients then have organic insulin pumps inside their bodies and never need to inject themselves again.

Genetic disorders

Currently, many gene therapies are used to cure diseases caused by specific genetic mutations. These therapies are often limited by the complexity of treatments and the constraints of transfection technologies. Thus, many of them target monogenic disorders, which are induced by the mutation of a single gene.

In our expectation, a Miao system is an upgraded gene delivery system that can be safely, efficiently, reliably, and repeatedly used. Such a system will greatly simplify the complicated procedures of gene therapies. In particular, once a level 3 Miao system is available, it may replace dangerous procedures such as spine injection with straightforward intramuscular injection. Moreover, there will be no more worry about serious antiviral immune responses and potential viral gene leftovers in the human genome. Hence, gene therapy may extend to more complicated multigenic diseases. Additionally, the capacity for repeated use of a Miao system always provides a second chance for patients.

No pain, no gain

The above examples illustrate the potential usage of Miao systems in treating diseases and disorders. These applications will be essential for reaching and maintaining HYL while reducing the odds of death for a long life. Such a system would support a larger lechatelierim to maintain the health and functions of the body.

A body that has never got sick is not healthy either. For example, like muscles, the immune system needs periodical "exercises" to recognize new antigens and increase efficiency. Although harmful and dangerous conditions should always be avoided, some gentle and controllable diseases could be made beneficial for our health. Similar to vaccination, the body may need to get through some harmless manmade diseases to strengthen its reactivity and cooperation between different organ systems. Therefore, gene delivery can be used to introduce mild antigens or create controlled conditions for the body to gradually increase its lechatelierim. However, LeChatelierism should always be followed to avoid substantial damage to the body.

The Enemies from Outside

When there is no enemy within, the enemy outside can do you no harm.
—African proverb

Viral, bacterial, fungal, and parasitic diseases are recorded in the first chapter of the *International Classification of Diseases*, which reflects their significant impacts on human health. Either seasonal flu or bacterial infection can become a lethal threat to people in HYL. Thus, as a critical part of task 3 in the roadmap (Figure 6), dealing with infectious diseases is essential for a long life.

A glimpse of a pandemic

If only one thing about 2020 is remembered by people in the future, it will be the COVID-19 pandemic caused by the severe acute respiratory syndrome coronavirus 2 (SARS-CoV-2). This virus rapidly spread around the globe, threatening every country and city. In less than a year, over 100 million people were infected, with over 2.5 million deaths worldwide.

As the world's leader with the highest standards of human healthcare and medicine, the United States had over 25 million cases of COVID-19. Cruise ships, nursing homes, bars, parties, and airports became concentration camps. Families, friends, and coworkers were infected, hospitalized, and even died together. The whole world was shocked by this pandemic. The economy was shattered, borders were closed, cities locked down, and many companies bankrupted. In the USA, the unemployment rate quadrupled and consumer spending dropped. Men and women waited for hours in front of food banks and the government sent money out to help people get through this hard time. The national debt soared while the stock market went crazy.

People no longer had their normal lives. Men and women put on face masks and kept social distances to avoid infection. Smiles were thus covered with fabrics. No more handshakes, no more lunch together, and no more intimate actions in public. Governments around the world issued lockdown orders to restrict the spread of the virus by keeping people at home. Adults worked at home, kids played at home, and families were trapped at home. Through the internet, people around the globe shared the same feeling of depression and uncertainty.

Healthcare workers and researchers responded quickly to the pandemic and fought hard against the coronavirus. The viral sequence was publicly available soon after the first observed case. Medical professionals worked hard to search for cures and develop therapies. A series of drugs were claimed to be effective against the virus, which led to an upsurge in the companies' stocks. However, the treatment results were ambiguous and the number of deaths continued to grow every day. Pharmaceutical companies and research institutes also pushed for the development of vaccines against SARS-CoV-2. Regulatory agencies from different countries shrank clinical trials from multiple years to several months. However, some reports indicated that immunity generated by vaccination could only last for less than a year. Nevertheless, in desperation and anxiety, people around the world still took the vaccines as their only hope to go back to normal. Unfortunately, the WHO predicted that the pandemic could accompany human beings for years and the world would probably *never* go back to what it used to be.

COVID-19 only took a few months to become the new No. 1 cause of death in the USA. Though bravely defending themselves, modern medicine and technology were quickly beaten up by a tiny virus. In this pandemic, human civilization swayed under the overwhelming power of Mother Nature.

Human beings strike back

In a 300-year life, a person is likely to meet several viral pandemics and many endemics. Most of them could be mild and quick, but a few may be lethal enough to reshape the world like the coronavirus outbreak. Surviving through the attack of a novel virus is a tough challenge.

When humans are the gladiators in the DNA master's arena, it is a matter of life or death and negligence can be fatal. Fortunately, modern medical technologies can quickly identify the virus and dissect its genome in days. The viral genetic information is our best way to know about the enemy so that we can develop suitable weapons against it. Therefore, scientists search in the book of life to look for a clue of death.

An appropriate Miao system can play an important role in fighting novel viruses. Gene delivery of ASOs can inhibit the expression of specific proteins. The ASO-induced suppression of gene expression is a mature technology with a high success rate. This can be accomplished by sending ASOs directly or through plasmids to express ASOs in cells. If the inhibited protein is critical for the proliferation of the virus, the inhibition prevents it from multiplication. Consequently, viral infection can be suppressed and blocked. A great advantage of such an antiviral strategy is that it can quickly react to viral outbreaks. Even if the virus is novel, the design of specific ASOs can be completed in a short period of time once the viral genetic information is available. The synthesis of ASOs or plasmids used for gene delivery usually takes days to weeks. Thus, before long, humans will have a prototypic weapon specifically against a novel virus. Of course, the efficacy and potential adverse effects of the ASOs need further testing, but they can always be easily modified and improved.

The required gene delivery system is comparatively simple

if the target is the lungs. The lungs are relatively exposed to the outside world and isolated from other parts of the body. This facilitates gene delivery but makes them more vulnerable. Many widespread viruses are airborne transmitted while quite a few attack and proliferate in the lungs. A series of gene therapies have been applied to the lungs for treating lung cancer and other serious lung diseases. Thus, a variety of gene delivery technologies have been used in the lungs and had impressive results. Although a level 3 Miao system is always preferred, a level 1 or even a level 0 Miao system may also be able to conduct gene delivery to transfect or express ASOs in the lungs. However, if the virus attacks other parts of the body, at least a level 2 Miao system should be used to eliminate the virus. Gene delivery can also activate other cellular pathways to facilitate the fight against the virus. Moreover, gene delivery can be used to suppress cytokine storms or other severe conditions caused by viral infections. The widespread use of gene delivery based antiviral procedures may block viral outbreaks at an early stage. In the COVID-19 pandemic, there were fewer than a thousand cumulative cases in the USA or the world within the first month of the outbreak. If the spread of the virus could have been stopped then, there would have been no pandemic. Millions of lives and trillions of dollars could thus have been saved.

Other than directly eliminating viruses, an appropriate Miao system can also be used for developing DNA or RNA vaccines. Traditional vaccines use live-attenuated or inactivated viruses, as well as recombinant viral proteins or protein fragments. The development and manufacturing of these vaccines take quite a long time. Moreover, some live-attenuated or inactivated viruses are still toxic or harmful to the human body. In contrast, DNA and RNA vaccines directly encode the genetic information about specific viral protein or protein fragments. After transfection, cells will synthesize the viral protein or protein fragments to initiate the immunogenetic process. The design and manufacture of DNA and RNA vaccines can be much faster than traditional vaccines. In the COVID-19 pandemic, the first vaccines used in the USA were RNA vaccines. With an appropriate Miao system, a candidate DNA or RNA vaccine can be quickly prepared and ready for testing. Although clinical trials still take time, the readiness of DNA and RNA vaccines makes them important weapons in the human arsenal against novel viral pandemics. If an emergency use authorization is issued, the manufacture of DNA and RNA vaccines can be rapidly scaled up for compulsory vaccination. This could be a savior for humankind.

The hidden enemies

Pathogenic bacteria, fungi, and parasites can live inside our bodies and cause serious diseases. Unlike viruses, they are alive and have their own life cycle. They utilize a series of mechanisms to protect themselves and survive in the human body. Current drugs mainly target specific proteins of these organisms. These drugs are difficult to develop and can be toxic to the human body. Meanwhile, more and more pathogens and parasites evolve resistance.

Many organisms have an active defense system against pathogens and parasites. Animals and plants generate a series of defensins, which are special peptides that only attack exogenous intruders without harming host cells. These small peptides vary in different animals and plants. They are effective against a wide spectrum of microbes and parasites. Insects also synthesize a group of proteins and peptides to cause inhibition at different stages of parasites' life cycle. This defense mechanism enables insects to coexist with parasites without being harmed.

In the human body, defensins are made only in specific immune cells. A strategy to defend the body against attacks from microbes and parasites is to conduct defensin gene delivery with an appropriate Miao system. Other than specific immune cells, many more cells can be induced to synthesize and secrete these defensive peptides. Therefore, the defense mechanism in the human body can be exponentially enhanced. Moreover, if not harmful to our bodies, genes of effective defensins from other species can be delivered to our cells, which can further facilitate the crackdown on intruders.

Another strategy for fighting against the invasion of pathogens and parasites is to deliver harmful genes to these organisms. One approach is to universally express specific proteins to suppress pathways that are unique to pathogenic organisms. This approach requires a suitable level 2 Miao system to cover all or most cells within the body, including all pathogenic and parasitic cells. Such an approach can be dangerous since human cells are also affected. Another approach is to conduct accurate gene delivery only to pathogens and parasites to damage them from inside. This approach is more difficult since it requires a level 3 Miao system to specifically target exogenous cells but not human cells. Nevertheless, either inhibiting vital microbial and parasitic genes or generating toxic substances in their cells should cause severe devastation to these intruders.

Forward to Basics

An apple a day keeps the doctor away.
—Welsh proverb

We have discussed disturbing conditions like infectious diseases and cancer. However, life is more about living safely and healthily each day. Thus, HYL always focuses on basics and details, which are tasks 1 and A in the roadmap (Figure 6).

Long and prosperous living

There are numerous philosophies and theories about living a healthy lifestyle. Despite the differences, most of them share a few time-honored ideas for maintaining a balanced and lasting life.

Know your body

Knowledge is power. All lifeforms are supported by information from the DNA master. If we would like to live beyond *Its* warranty, we need to know how to sustain ourselves.

There are so many books about the human body, but we don't need to be as knowledgeable as physicians or scientists. However, understanding the basics of the human body updates our common sense to keep it logical and realistic. It prevents the potential idiocy that causes us big trouble and ruins our path to HYL. For example, in the COVID-19 pandemic, some Americans drank bleach in an attempt to kill the coronavirus. They still ended up in the emergency room, but not for viral infection. Similarly, some people believe that eating raw meat from wild animals brings them strength and vigor. However, what they usually get instead are happy parasites that feast on a buffet inside their bodies. In both examples, those people believe they are doing the right thing based on their knowledge of the human body. Unfortunately, their understanding is not grounded in the basic rules of biology and chemistry. These examples are quite extreme and some people would think that they cannot be deceived that easily. How about a month-long fasting program recommended by a famous health guru, or a high-tech superfood claimed to cure all diseases? Many people have believed similar things and paid their price. Knowing more about the human body helps us avoid being fooled by others or by our own minds.

You are what you eat

There are countless diet tips and recipes on the internet. It is easy to know why. Food keeps us alive by providing nutrients and energy that are essential for our bodies. Food also produces simple yet delightful satisfaction. Thus, everyone likes delicious food and we always need to feed ourselves several times a day. Fortunately, there are innumerable kinds of ingredients and cooking methods. Therefore, people around the world find various ways to eat healthily and happily.

Most healthy eating tips aim to reach a balanced food intake in the long term. The general advice is not to eat too much or too little to keep the body in a harmonious state. Also, many recommendations advocate eating less. This advice is quite against human nature. With thousands of years of starving memories engraved in our genes, our bodies naturally want to greedily devour any food we can find. Thanks to modern agriculture, food supply is no longer a problem for many of us. However, the specter of sugar addiction is still haunting us. In this case, if we follow our nature, we will likely get a big belly and have a sky-high body mass index (BMI). If we are lucky, we will also receive diabetes, heart problems, fatty liver, damaged kidneys, rotten teeth, and other more surprising gifts. Our bodies just haven't adapted to the world of mechanized farming and industrialized food production. Even in the next millennium, the human body probably won't get used to having so many available foods. Some problems caused by eating too much can be relieved or even solved with a suitable Miao system. However, the best and simplest solution is that we wisely choose our energy intake. Some people recommend taking a fasting day every few weeks or conducting intermittent fasting. These practices follow the habit of our bodies, mimicking what our ancestors experienced for thousands of years. Thus, such lifestyles are believed to boost and maintain health. Those statements are also supported by results from some molecular studies. A lot of DNA damage is caused by ROS, many of which are produced from the foods we eat. Consequently, the more food intake, the more ROS, and thus more DNA damage that could lead to cancer. More nutrients and energy also facilitate cell replication, which results in shortened telomeres. Besides, many food byproducts can burden the heart and disrupt the hormone system. Therefore, despite the tastiness, some foods are less healthy than others and have thus been called "junk" food.

Another almost universal healthy eating tip is to have a balanced diet. Carbohydrates with fibers, proteins, healthy fats, vitamins, minerals, and antioxidants are all essential for a healthy life. Various kinds of food ingredients, which are composed of these nutrients, are sweet gifts to us from the DNA master for prolonging *Its* existence. We should gladly accept the rewards and enjoy them happily to celebrate our survival.

Nowadays, many people choose to avoid certain kinds of food because of personal, lifestyle, cultural, or religious reasons. As long as a full spectrum of nutrition is supplied, such a choice doesn't have a great impact on health. However, it is a pity if the body is compromised due to nutrition deficiency. The appropriate ratio between different nutrients has been argued about for a long time and is largely affected by culture. Governments around the world have created food pyramids and other charts as recommendations for food intake. Since the standards used are biased towards the habits of the country's population, the directions vary accordingly. For example, the recommendation for Chinese people has much more vegetables and less meat. Because of the many variations, it is difficult to identify the world's best food pyramid. Based on life expectancy, some people think the Okinawa diet developed by the inhabitants of that Japanese island is the healthiest diet plan. People in Okinawa had the longest life expectancy in Japan for many years, while Japan has the highest life expectancy of all countries. Interestingly, the life expectancy of Okinawans has dropped since they switched to Westernized food. Thus, some people believe the Okinawa diet is their secret to longevity. However, such a diet may not be suitable for everyone. It is difficult to determine if the same result can be reproduced without the local food and lifestyle. Due to the diversity of human culture and lifestyle, the best diet plan in the world will remain an open question for a long time. Nevertheless, maintaining a balanced diet is always a good strategy.

Run for your health

"Exercise regularly" is another universal piece of health advice. Nowadays, almost all experts believe that regular exercise makes the body fit and healthy.

The opinion about exercise has changed over time. Although human beings made it to the peak of the evolutionary tree by using the brain, the worship of the body began while our ancestors were still among the animals. In the early days, more muscle gave people more power to throw a spear or an arrow and thus take down a deer or a rabbit. Muscle power directly correlated to the amount of meat a hunter brought back to his or her family and tribe. Even for gatherers, more power meant a person could carry home more baskets of fruits and vegetables. Moreover, a tougher body could help people get through difficult times like pregnancy or starvation. Therefore, physical strength has been worshiped since then. People with powerful bodies were portrayed as gods and heroes in ancient mythologies.

However, things changed after people settled for agriculture. Persistence became a more important trait than strength for growing food to feed the family. Moreover, feudal governments preferred people with compliant natures since that made the job of ruling easier. Indeed, muscular men and women have more physical power to oppose authority. More muscles are also associated with steroids, which could give people the impulse to engage in rebellious activities. Thus, in some cultures, physical strength was no longer worshiped as much as before. This is especially true for many Asian countries that were influenced by Confucianism. These countries believed that obedience is one of the top virtues of civilization. For this reason, military officials were even officially discriminated against by other officials for hundreds of years. During certain extreme times, overweight men and underweight women were fashionable. This is because such body types indicated that these people had prosperous lives and didn't have to work miserably in the fields, raising crops. Lacking exercise, these people were not suited to any kind of physical activity, including military operations. Consequently, these countries were at a great disadvantage in the many wars that occurred with nomads from the north.

Later, the Renaissance aroused people's worship of the beauty of the human body. Thus, body curves and strong muscles became trendy again. After the Industrial Revolution, many people were freed from endless manual labor. As a result, a fit body tuned from exercise has become a way to show a person's lifestyle and social status. It implies an expensive gym membership with personal trainers, a house large enough for a treadmill and other gear, or free time and money spent on exercise and sports. Nevertheless, regular exercise does bring a lot of benefits to the human body.

The amount of exercise required for fitness has been under

debate. More exercise does not always lead to a healthier body. For example, professional athletes have much more exercise than average people. However, many of them suffer injuries, pain, and other conditions, even years after they retire. Some athletes also take performance-enhancing drugs to obtain more strength, agility, or focus. However, many of these drugs are risky with serious adverse effects. For example, some commonly used steroids can lead to severe acne, depression, high blood pressure, and even heart attack. Even some popular exercises can cause body damage. For example, running the 26.2-mile marathon is a trendy sport for runners around the world. As a great physical challenge, it pushes the body to its limit. Knee and muscle injuries are common among runners and adverse effects on the heart and kidney have also been reported. Moreover, prolonged metabolism increase with large oxygen consumption creates a lot of ROS that can cause DNA damage. Therefore, it is hard to determine if the benefits of such sports outweigh the side effects.

In contrast, some people have too little exercise. Most of their physical activities are limited to their hands: using cellphones or playing video games. Low levels of exercise have been known to be harmful to health. They can lead to obesity, heart disease, Type II diabetes, and some types of cancer.

A reasonable strategy for maintaining our health is a balance between these extreme examples. Some experts suggest keeping BMI between 18 and 25 by diet and exercise. Conducting 30 minutes or more of intermediate exercise three to five times a week is recommended. If the same routine was kept throughout a 300-year life, it would be equivalent to years spent in the gym. If a Miao system is sophisticated enough, we can use it to adjust our metabolism and hormone levels. It is thus possible to mimic the effects of exercise without going to the gym. If this happens in the future, it would be interesting to see if people still take time to exercise when everyone has a perfect body.

Small things, big impact

Our habits accompany us throughout our lives. Therefore, even for a trivial routine, repeating it daily for 300 years can have a huge effect on us.

For example, sleep disorders and related problems bother a lot of people. Insomnia is becoming more common since people work longer hours and the brain remains active late at night. Having a few hours' less sleep does not seem to be a big deal. However, for a 300-year life, that would be 20–30 years of lost rest and recovery time for the body. Insomnia not only causes fatigue and depression but also increases the risk of reduced brain performance and accidents. Moreover, it induces many diseases and disorders, such as obesity, weak immune system, high blood pressure, heart disease, and stroke. Therefore, a good night's sleep is important for a person's health. Many sleeping pills have been commercialized to treat insomnia. However, side effects such as headache, dizziness, and addiction are their common problems. If gene delivery can be frequently and easily used, the melatonin level in the body can be readily adjusted to facilitate sleep so that the body can sufficiently recover from tiredness and damage.

Personal hygiene also has a big impact on health. Infectious diseases pose a major threat to human lives, but the chance of infection can be dramatically reduced by maintaining good personal hygiene. For example, it has been reported that handwashing can reduce the risk of respiratory infections by 16%. Some researchers estimate that a million deaths a year could be prevented if everyone routinely washed his or her hands. Many infectious diseases are more lethal to older people and immunocompromised persons. In the COVID-19 pandemic, 80% of deaths occur in people 65 years old and above. The death rate of people who are 80 years old and above is over 70 times higher than people who are 30 years old and younger. Thus, before the body is rejuvenated, infectious diseases can be a primary peril to a long life. The risk of SARS-CoV-2 infection can be dramatically reduced by simply wearing a high-quality facemask and frequent hand sanitation. Many infectious diseases can be prevented in the same way. Therefore, keeping good personal hygiene saves lives.

Keep out of trouble

The secret of life is to maintain balance: keep disturbances within the lechatelierim so that the situation is always under control. Otherwise, no matter in normal life or HYL, the path to death can be an expedited one-way ticket. Hence, LeChatelierism is fundamental for a hyper-long life. Even if the body is rejuvenated and immune to diseases, a person can still be easily killed by a crashing car or burning fire. Therefore, avoiding danger is of extreme importance and is listed as task 1 in the roadmap (Figure 6).

Risk factors that can cause sudden death or great damage to the body should always be avoided. It could be a war, a riot, a street fight, a house on fire, a car with bad brakes, a cobra at large, a hairdryer in a filled bathtub, a wrong choice of medicine, a cup of polluted water, a slippery ladder, or anything else. Accidents happen, so a long life is never guaranteed. Our primitive animal instinct enables us to detect and react to hazards around us. This sense is further enhanced by years of nagging from our parents and learning from our own experiences. However, danger always lures us with the promise of excitement and tricks us into believing that we can win the game of probability. Those are the moments to pay extra attention to.

Risk factors for chronic harm are more deceptive than immediate dangers. A common example is smoking, which can cause cancer, heart disease, stroke, lung diseases, and diabetes. Toxins trapped in the lungs cannot be removed, leading to years of continuous damage. Smoking on average shortens life expectancy by over 10 years. Despite all the serious adverse effects, one in seven people smokes. Consequently, smoking is responsible for 8 million annual deaths worldwide. Alcohol abuse is similar. Any alcohol intake, as little as a single glass of beer, creates DNA damage and increases the risk of cancer. Along with other acute and long-term toxic effects of alcohol, taking only one drink a day shortens life expectancy by a year.

A basic function of human intellect is to plan for long-term benefits. Unlike other animals, we are willing to give up short-term satisfaction for a better future. Thus, humans collect seeds for sowing, put lures in traps, store foods for winter, go to university for career development, hold stocks for gains, and save money for retirement. Evaluating and following long-term benefits makes us stand out from the animal kingdom. Civilization developed in this way, as well as wars, religions, investments, liars, insurance companies, and advanced degrees. Considering the long term is essential for making smart decisions.

Drug addiction blocks this important logical circuit with chemical stimulants. The glory of human intellect is overshadowed by moments of overwhelmingly strong ecstasy. Drug use triggers the reward system in the brain with positive feedbacks to gradually enslave the consciousness. Legal or not, this is a sweet yet treacherous deathtrap. Drugs are associated with numerous serious conditions: cancer, asthma, bronchitis, emphysema, nausea, vomiting, dehydration, abdominal pain, infectious diseases like HIV and hepatitis, overall muscle weakness, paranoia, depression, anxiety, and many more. These conditions are great threats to both normal life and HYL.

The world is full of tradeoffs and people need to choose wisely on the path to HYL. Stepping into the dark side won't lead to a happy long life.

Little bits here and there
Health is not just about the body. Mental health is as critical

as physical health. Thus, it is always important to keep a positive mindset filled with joy, hope, confidence, optimism, and kindness. We are also affected by things around us. A safe environment creates serenity of the mind, helping the body to maintain its balance. Moreover, a sweet love life, strong family connection, and favorable social support are also beneficial for HYL.

109,500 times

Life is a long journey. A 300-year life is an even longer voyage with 109,500 sunrises and sunsets to experience. We can take only one small step each day to cover the distance. In this journey, persistence is the key to reaching the finish line.

Shortcuts

People have been seeking rejuvenation and longevity for many thousands of years and will continue to do so in the future. This book is also a part of this ongoing mission.

The charm of *longevity pills* is irresistible. They have made many appearances throughout human history. In the early days, longevity pills were religious relics, supernatural artifacts, alchemic essences, or exotic precious stones. When modern medicine was developed, acetylsalicylic acid and vitamin C became the new legends. Later, longevity pills became sirolimus, metformin, nicotinamide riboside, or the trendy senolytics. On each occasion, longevity pills are at the frontier of knowledge of that time. Their power has been continuously worshiped and many of them do have certain beneficial effects on the human body.

Searching for a longevity pill is quite a good business. With such an attractive subject, it is not difficult to obtain investment. The legends of Xu Fu from China and Juan Ponce de León from Spain are still popular. Nowadays, the most engaging opening would be an eye-catching theory or concept, even better when the team has a renowned professor on board. Longevity research is always a long-term investment. Drug screening is time-consuming; it can take years, followed by multiple rounds of redesign and development. Thus, the team needs to be fed on investors' money for quite a while. The evaluation of longevity drugs usually takes longer than normal drugs. For mice studies, researchers probably need to wait until the end of the mice's lifespan, which lasts several years and could even be extended. Similar trials on humans can take even longer. Theoretically, the best evaluation should last until the end of the hopefully extended lifespan of the subjects. This is not practical for obvious reasons.

Time is money. Thus, losing time, at least to some people, is losing money. Following the usual pattern, if a reasonably promising outcome was found in mice, the longevity pill would be readily commercialized. Human testing doesn't always seem necessary in the business world and, in several cases, successful commercialization has been achieved based only on results in mice. A smart approach could be promoting natural compounds that are already present in the body in large amounts. These compounds are generally safe, have known beneficial effects, are easy to produce on a large scale, and are usually well-received by the public. Therefore, online stores are filled with numerous kinds of bottles of white tablets with "longevity" printed on the package. Moreover, tens of thousands of webpages are loaded with articles suggesting that one of these tablets is the savior of the future of humankind.

People's simple hope for longevity thus is transformed into valuable "ka-ching" sounds. As a result, everyone is happy: investors, researchers, laboratory renters, instrument sellers, maintenance engineers, mouse keepers, pill manufacturers, bottle makers, box packers, advertisement designers, online store managers, internet providers, webpage writers, mail carriers, buyers who spend the money, buyers' spouses who take the pills to feel younger, and tax collectors. This is a wonderful world.

At the beginning of this book, we discussed how unlikely it is that we will find a single or a few compounds that can dramatically extend the human lifespan. The human body is a sophisticated machine, which consists of complicated and intertwined systems. Different aspects of the body are coordinated and maintained by distinct yet similar mechanisms. There *might* exist one thing to rule them all, but the possibility is exceptionally tiny.

Currently, many longevity pills target one of the essential pathways, such as suppressing ROS, reducing DNA damage, inhibiting specific receptors, activating cells, and boosting immunity. As demonstrated in previous chapters, each of these mechanisms only covers a limited part of human health. The improvement of only one or a few aspects of the body is not enough to extend human life much beyond its natural boundary. For example, a person with enhanced antibacterial immunity but normal anticancer mechanisms is not likely to live much longer than a person with normal antibacterial immunity and normal anticancer mechanisms. Their chances of getting and dying of cancer should be quite similar. These two examples are fairly common in the population, but neither of them has lived 150 years. However, if one aspect of health is deficient, it may easily compromise the beneficial effects of all other aspects. It can even become deadly. For example, a person with enhanced antibacterial immunity but deficient anticancer mechanisms is likely to live a shorter life than a person with normal antibacterial immunity and normal anticancer mechanisms. The first person has a much higher chance of getting and dying of cancer, which trims his or her life expectancy. Therefore, even if one or a few compounds could enhance one or a few essential pathways, it is unlikely to dramatically improve overall health and largely extend lifespan. Since so many aspects of health need to be covered, there are a series of tasks in the roadmap for reaching and maintaining HYL (Figure 6).

Figure 10.
2D molecular structures of vitamin C (left)
and vitamin B$_{12}$ (right).

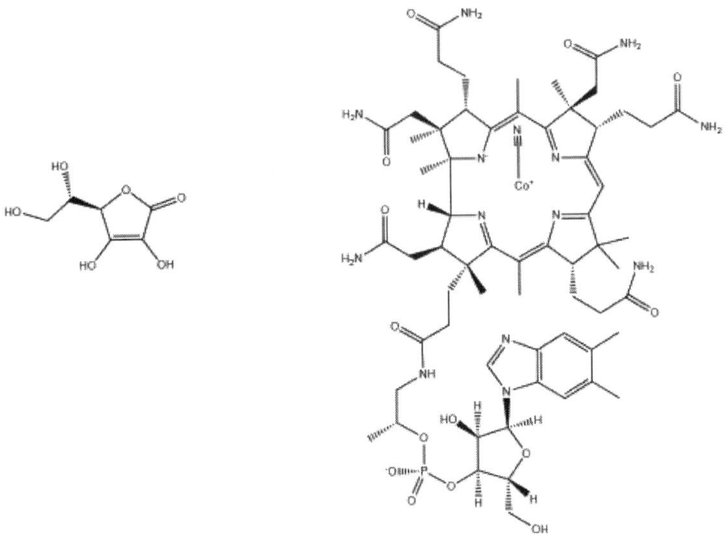

Vitamin C (L-ascorbic acid)   Vitamin B$_{12}$ (cobalamin)

Even if one or a few compounds could target *all* the essential health pathways, it is extremely difficult for them to have enough specificity for *each* of the pathways. The reason is simple: enzymes in those pathways are very diverse. Biochemical reactions in our bodies are catalyzed by enzymes with distinct structures to recognize numerous molecules through direct interactions. For example, vitamin C (L-ascorbic acid) and vitamin B$_{12}$ (cobalamin) are common cofactors of different enzymes in the body (Figure 10). These two compounds are so dissimilar that they cannot both be *specifically* recognized by

122

the same binding site of an enzyme. Likewise, the specificity of different enzymes cannot be fulfilled by a single compound. Given that there are thousands of kinds of enzymes in the human body, it is extremely unlikely that one or a few compounds can specifically interact with many of these enzymes and lead to beneficial effects in all the essential pathways.

Let us assume that someone has created a longevity pill that contains all the required compounds to improve all the important health pathways for extending lifespan. However, such a longevity pill probably won't work on all of us. The diversity of the body is huge and the required amount for each compound can vary dramatically for different people. For example, steak is many people's favorite food since it is delicious and provides a lot of proteins. However, steak can be poisonous for people with phenylketonuria since that amount of protein may induce brain damage. Metabolism varies greatly even between healthy people. For example, some people can easily withstand sugar shock from high-sugar foods but some people would develop diabetes. Therefore, even if a longevity pill was created, it could be difficult to find a universal dose for everyone. If personalized therapy is required for cancer treatment, how could taking a tablet a day solve the longevity problem for everyone?

Moreover, the positive effects induced by a longevity pill may not be beneficial in the long term, especially when the pill only activates a specific receptor. For a bidirectional lechatelierim, cells require both positive and negative feedbacks to maintain their balance. If the signal is always positive, it creates constant stimulations that could shift the balance to one direction and break the lechatelierim. For example, Ras is a family of essential proteins that are conserved in all animals. When Ras is switched on by external signals, it activates other proteins for cell proliferation and differentiation. Therefore, Ras is vital for cell survival. However, a mutated Ras that is always *on* is a total disaster. It constantly sends positive signals to the cell and pushes it to proliferate. Consequently, the cell could become cancerous. Mutated Ras is found in about 25% of all human cancers. In some cancer types, 90% of the patients have Ras mutations. Likewise, if a longevity pill constantly provides positive signals to cells, it could lead to unpredicted adverse results in the long term. Always good isn't always good.

Many longevity pills have shown efficacy in mice and thus have been commercialized. Even if we assume mice and humans share the same metabolism, the human lifespan is 30 times longer than that of mice. Thus, many effects during such a long time cannot be evaluated by studying rodents. For example, sustained receptor activation could cause the marginal utility of the longevity pill to diminish. This means that the effect of new pills may decrease if too many pills have been taken. The law of diminishing marginal utility was first developed in economics to describe the benefit derived by consuming a product. It has also been applied to many fields of science. A typical example in biology is drug addiction. Many abused drugs have diminishing marginal utility. Consequently, people who do drugs have to take more and more drugs to reach the same level of stimulation. Similarly, if a longevity pill has diminishing marginal utility, increased daily intake is required to reach the same level of beneficial effect. After decades of continuous use, the required daily amount could be extremely high and addiction to the longevity pill could develop. The body may also evolve mechanisms to adapt to the high concentration of pills in it. If this is the case, any disruption to the continuous intake could suddenly disturb metabolism, which could lead to serious adverse effects.

Therefore, the existence of true longevity pills and other simple solutions for rejuvenation and longevity is questionable. Even if they exist, they are probably not as desirable as people expect. Hence, a reasonable strategy is to admire the complexity of life and treat it as such. As demonstrated in previous chapters, the diamond drill worshiped in this book is a platform technology that can be widely used in a series of tasks and scenarios to reach and maintain HYL. Even though a level 3 Miao system is very powerful, there are still many tasks that it cannot accomplish, and these would have to be completed by other methodologies. Some tasks can be achieved by other technologies, such as organ transplantation; some tasks can be dealt with by ourselves, such as keeping a healthy lifestyle; some tasks are in the hands of the universe and we cannot do anything about them. Complicated as it is, *c'est la vie*.

There is no shortcut to HYL. However, by learning, doing, and repeating the basics, we will increase our odds of success.

Neurons: A New Frontier

You are nothing but a pack of neurons.
—Francis Crick

The nervous system, which includes the brain where our ego resides, is still quite mysterious to us. Luckily, on our path to HYL, we don't need to worry about the nervous system for a long time: neurons live longer than we can live.

The apex of the human body

Our brain is astonishingly magnificent. As the pearl of biology, it represents the summit of 3.8 billion years of evolution. There are about 100 billion neurons in the brain, which is similar in number to stars in the Milky Way galaxy. These neurons form over 100 thousand miles of nerve fibers, which is more than enough to surround Earth four times. Moreover, these neurons create over 150 trillion neural connections, or synapses, with one another. This number is 75 times the number of galaxies in the observable universe. In this massive network, neurons transmit information by electrochemical impulses with speeds up to 120 m/s (268 mph), which is faster than most cars. The billions of neurons are supported by ten times more cells called glia. Glial cells assist neurons to migrate to their designated positions and hold them in place. They also surround neurons to protect them, supply nutrients, facilitate neurotransmission, and destroy pathogens. Together, neurons and glia build the massive network of the nervous system. The brain is the powerful CPU of this system. It conducts incredible calculations, flights of imagination, and thinking, in which consciousness is born. Even the most advanced supercomputer hasn't been able to replicate all the functions of 150 trillion synapses in the brain. As mighty as it is, the brain operates with only about 10 watts of energy, which is much more energy-efficient than most personal computers. With this unbelievably powerful machine, the fragile apes have written a new chapter of Earth's history. Every great achievement in human civilization is initiated by simple electrochemical sparks in someone's brain. Therefore, the brain is undoubtedly the DNA master's most sophisticated masterpiece. These invaluable treasures are sitting peacefully in our heads.

Out from the brain come 12 pairs of cranial nerves and the spinal cord, which connects to different parts of the body via 31 pairs of spinal nerves. These nerves consist of billions of neurons of mainly three types: sensory neurons, motor neurons, and interneurons. They intertwine to form a complex network of nerves and ganglia to sense various signals from different parts of the body and pass them to the brain. After the information is processed by the brain, the nerves pass the orders from the brain to the body parts to control motions and reactions. The nervous system is thus a sophisticated communication network that keeps the body functioning properly.

Neurons are the longest-living cells in our bodies. Most of them were already existing when we were born, while limited neurogenesis occurs throughout our lives. Many cells in the human body are replaced periodically. For example, some neutrophils only survive for hours. However, neurons can last a lifetime. Unlike most other cells in our bodies, neurons do not replicate or proliferate. Without damage and disease, the neuron lifespan is only limited by how long their host, such as us, can live. Neurons can last even longer than their host. In an experiment, Dr. Ferdinando Rossi transplanted mouse neural precursor cells into the brains of rats. The mouse neurons developed and lived normally in rat brains until the death of the rats. Since rats have a lifespan that is twice as long as that of mice, the mouse neurons lived much longer than the mice they were from. Similarly, if our neurons have an environment conducive to their survival, they will continue to live after the passing away of us. The longest-living mammals, bowhead whales, can live 200–300 years. Therefore, mammalian neurons should be able to survive 300 years without too much trouble. Hence, 300 years is selected as the target age in this book as our goal of HYL.

Androids, clones, and cyborgs

All our ego and consciousness is in the nervous system, more specifically, the central nervous system (the brain and spinal cord). If neurons can live longer than the rest of the body, why not just preserve the nervous system, or only the brain, to keep our thinking and memories? These are trendy hypothetical approaches to accomplish longevity or even eternity.

Mind uploading is one of these exciting concepts, in which the molecular status and electrochemical signals of a brain are scanned and copied to a computer. The computer then simulates the functions of the scanned brain to replicate the same thinking logic and processes. The computer could control an android or other robots so that the uploaded brain would have a body. Alternatively, it could remain as an isolated device like a normal computer. To reach this goal, neurobiologists and computer scientists have developed a series of technologies. For example, functional magnetic resonance imaging (fMRI) and electroencephalogram scanners record various signals from the brain, while machine learning and neural network algorithms artificially mimic thinking procedures. These technologies have already had vast impacts on the healthcare industry as well as our daily life. However, it is still unlikely that our minds can be precisely uploaded to computers in the foreseeable future. Current human technology is not even close to having the resolution and accuracy to identify, separate, and record the specific states of the 100 billion neurons in the human brain. This is only the prerequisite for monitoring and understanding the statuses of 150 trillion synapses. To get detailed information from all the neurons, examining the brain from outside may not be sufficient. One possible approach is to physically separate the brain into a series of ultra-thin slices for detailed scanning and analyses. However, this will lead to irreversible damage to the brain of the examinee and the end of his or her life.

The enormous complexity of the brain will create a tremendous amount of data upon scanning. Even if each synapse only has the two states of "on" and "off," recording an instance of all synapses in the brain would generate at least 19 terabytes of data. Differences in neuronal microenvironments contribute to various combinations of compound composition, concentration, and local voltage at individual synapses. Since each synapse has numerous states, data generated by 150 trillion synapses can be enormously huge. However, this provides only a snapshot of the brain; it is far from replicating its intelligence. Thinking is more of a process than a state. Looking at photos of Chinese people cannot enable us to speak Mandarin. Similarly, one instance of the brain cannot reflect all the excellencies of its functions. Moreover, parts of the thinking processes are randomly determined by real-time synaptic states. It would be challenging to identify and extract such randomness from a snapshot of the brain. Therefore, even if the scanning of a brain is completed, the reconstruction of the thinking process could still be difficult. Since capturing only one snapshot may require the breakup of a brain, obtaining enough instances of the same brain to mimic its thinking processes could be almost impossible.

Human self-awareness is spontaneously developed through thinking processes. Children realize that they are individual entities not because their parents have told them so. Instead, they find out that they are unique objects by living and interacting with the rest of the world. However, such natural processes cannot be replicated to create human self-awareness after uploading information from a brain. The computer engineer may input some parameters to command the virtual brain to start "thinking" that it is someone. The virtual brain then may *appear* to be self-aware. However, does the virtual brain act like a person because it truly has self-awareness, or is it just the mindless output of a scripted function associated with its particular datatype? The latter is still a brainless dummy, no matter how real it behaves. To create a dull simulator doesn't seem to be worth the risks of dissecting a brain.

Mind uploading could be by transfer or copying. Either way, what would happen to the body and the brain? Is the original mind destroyed during the scan or deleted afterward? Abandoning ego and life just to complete a piece of computer software doesn't seem a wise choice. Even if the brain is not harmed during mind uploading, there will likely exist at least two copies of the same mind. "How to deal with another me?" will become a complicated problem. Chances are, the virtual person is thinking something similar.

If we cannot upload our minds to computers, how about preserving the nervous system after the body is worn out? It could be transferred to a cloned body, an incubator, or other suitable containers. This approach could be difficult to achieve. The nervous system is tangled up with the rest of the body by millions of nerves. It would be enormously challenging to separate all the tiny connections between neurons and other cells, especially when the body is still alive. Damage to neurons seems inevitable and it can be extremely painful if the sensory neurons are injured. If the nervous system is transferred to a cloned body, the reverse process has to be conducted to link the neurons with the new body, which doubles the challenges. However, neurons may not survive or function properly without the indigenous cells around them. So far, the original host body is still the only device that can sustain and support the nervous system.

Instead of preserving the whole nervous system, some scientists have suggested preserving only the brain, maybe with the head and parts of the spinal cord. Some researchers have even conducted experiments to transfer the head of one animal to another. However, the results are not promising. Even for animals of the same species, current technology cannot functionally connect spinal cords from different individuals. Those test animals died miserably, paralyzed. Therefore, it would be extremely difficult to install our heads on others' bodies or our clones to extend life.

In some sci-fi movies, the brain is taken out and incubated in special containers. This seems a good solution if a functional brain could be healthily maintained for a long time. However, the brain and the person in it probably won't have any privacy. Whatever the brain thinks will be transparent to at least the supporting staff members. It could be very embarrassing to disclose one's deepest and most detailed thoughts to others, totally naked to the brain. Besides, an incubated brain is very fragile and vulnerable. It could be easily damaged by a small power failure of the incubator. If someone hacks the brain and implants malware that simulates endless tortures and pains, it would be much worse than death.

An alternative strategy is to embed chips onto or into the brain. The chips could be used to sense brain activities and possibly enhance brain functions. Such technologies have been developed for many years and applied to certain animals and even humans, though there are still many concerns.

One challenge is to precisely translate thoughts from brain signals. Currently, fMRI and other technologies can sense some basic emotions and feelings. They have been used for developing devices to help disabled people. However, these technologies still cannot translate basic daily thoughts such as "I want to have a yummy double cheeseburger with crispy fried onion rings for lunch at the restaurant on 56th Avenue after this tedious conference call." In an ideal world or sci-fi movies, the chip on or in the brain understands this thought and makes a reservation at the restaurant. This is fantastically cool, though letting a chip and the company behind it examine the deepest secrets of the brain seems terrifying. However, even with further development of current technologies, the complete and accurate translation of human thoughts is not promising. The reason is simple. As previously described, thinking is conducted by millions of neurons, whose individual signals cannot be constantly monitored by these technologies with enough resolution. Thus, the signals the chip receives always lack parts of, if not most of, the information. This makes accurate reconstruction and translation difficult. Probes embedded inside the brain could probably improve resolution, though tracing the signals of single neurons is still implausible. Moreover, inserting a chip or an electrode into the brain seems scary and risky.

Enhancing brain functions using a chip can also be dangerous. Such technologies aim to coordinate brain neurons to make more use of the body. For example, it could increase power, agility, or memory by stimulating specific parts of the brain. This is very fascinating but it may not be as good as it seems. Many of our senses and feelings, such as pain, are calibrated specifically to our bodies. They identify dangers and restrict body movements for our protection. If such mechanisms are suppressed by a chip or other devices, we could ignore hazards or accidentally use more force than the body can bear. Consequently, we could leave foreign objects in our eye, run too fast and tear our leg muscles, or push the door too hard and break our forearm. Moreover, brainwashing is always a concern. Our brainwaves can be affected and hindered by external electromagnetic waves. The chip on or in the brain could undetectably shift our decisions or behaviors. For example, it could intentionally push a person to cast a wrong vote, or unintentionally make a person wet his or her pants during a software upgrade. If letting a chip and the company behind it read the deepest secrets of a person's brain seems terrifying, letting them operate his or her brain and body will scare the goosebumps out of him or her. Or maybe not, since his or her body and goosebumps are already controlled by the chip and the company behind it.

Therefore, due to the complexity of the nervous system, reaching and maintaining HYL seems a simpler and more practical approach to extend the existence of our minds. At least it has succeeded in many animals without manipulating their brains.

The vulnerable

Although neurons live a very long time, they can still be damaged and killed. For example, a stroke can break the oxygen and nutrient supply in the brain, causing the deaths of many neurons and brain damage. Since the brain is the headquarters of the body, its damage can lead to severe adverse effects and even death. Nerve injuries outside the brain can also have serious consequences. For example, spinal cord injury can break the communication between nearby neurons, which can cause paralysis such as hemiplegia. Therefore, neural maintenance is important for HYL and is listed as task D in the roadmap (Figure 6).

If a neuron is completely severed, it may not recover. This is particularly true for the central nervous system, where neuronal growth is very slow and likely inhibited by surrounding cells. A level 1 Miao system could probably suppress the inhibition and induce the growth of damaged neurons. However, it is still unclear if these neurons could recover successfully. The reestablishment of synapses may require more detailed adjustments that are beyond the current understanding of neurogenesis. Moreover, due to the complexity of the nervous system, it has been impossible so far to replace injured human neurons with functionally similar ones. Therefore, even if neurons are regenerated outside the body, neuron transplantation may not recover the damaged function. Hence, "prevention is better than cure" is especially true for the nervous system. Avoiding danger and keeping a healthy lifestyle to reduce potential neural injuries and damage are particularly important.

Besides direct injuries, neurons gradually lose their functions or are killed in various neurodegenerative processes. These processes can generate serious damage to the nervous system, causing neurodegenerative diseases such as Alzheimer's disease, Parkinson's disease, and Huntington's disease. Patients with these diseases gradually lose control of their bodies, which eventually leads to death. Such terrible diseases are still incurable. Many treatments only relieve the symptoms and barely slow down the progress of the disease. These neurodegenerative diseases are huge challenges for reaching and maintaining HYL. However, the exact causes and mechanisms of many of these diseases are still unclear, which creates obstacles to the development of specific therapies.

Alzheimer's disease and Parkinson's disease are the most common neurodegenerative diseases; each impairs millions of patients around the world. Both diseases are related to neuronal deaths in the brain. In Alzheimer's disease, neurons that regulate memory receive the largest impact, which causes dementia. Patients also progressively lose the ability to do everyday tasks. In Parkinson's disease, neurons that control body movements are mainly affected. Thus, symptoms usually start with hand tremors and loss of balance. The exact causes of both Alzheimer's disease and Parkinson's disease are unknown. Therefore, it is difficult to prevent and cure neurodegeneration in these diseases. Neuronal deaths in both diseases are related to abnormal accumulation of different proteins. However, whether these proteins directly cause cell death or are parts of cellular protective mechanisms is still debatable. A level 3 Miao system could conduct gene delivery to possibly remove the abnormal accumulated proteins, but it is unclear whether this could help cure the diseases. Many other neurodegenerative diseases also involve abnormal protein accumulations in brain neurons, such as Creutzfeldt-Jakob disease caused by infectious prions, Pick's disease, and diffuse Lewy body disease.

Some neurodegenerative diseases are caused by inherited genetic disorders. One example is Huntington's disease, which is caused by the expansion of repeated DNA sequences in the huntingtin gene. It results in mutated proteins that induce neuronal death in the brain. The patients suffer from uncoordinated movements caused by brain damage. The development of Huntington's disease progressively and irreversibly leads to death. The disease-causing DNA repeats in the huntingtin gene are like a molecular clock. They expand throughout the patient's lifetime and across generations when the genome is passed to the person's children. Once the repeated sequence achieves certain lengths, the disease initiates. Therefore, people with the expanding repeats or their descendants will eventually develop Huntington's disease. This cruel mechanism is like a time bomb deployed by the DNA master. Since Huntington's disease is caused by a single gene, modifying or suppressing the mutant gene should prevent or reverse the development of the disease. However, with current technology, it is difficult to conduct gene therapies to the whole brain and delete the long repeats. A suitable level 3 Miao system will likely be required for this task.

Some single gene neurodegenerative diseases are currently treatable using gene therapy. For example, spinal muscular atrophy is treated by injecting ASOs. It is one of the most expensive therapies in the world and each injection costs over

$100,000. The patients have to take spinal injections every four months throughout their lifetime. Despite the high cost, disease symptoms can be greatly relieved. In contrast, there is still no cure for most neurodegenerative diseases caused by multiple genes or unknown factors. Detailed molecular understanding of these diseases and a suitable Miao system will be essential for defeating these diseases in the future.

Trek beyond

When people say they want to live longer, usually their true meaning is to extend the existence of their consciousness. The body can be easily preserved for a very long time if it is immersed in formaldehyde or frozen in liquid nitrogen. A person can also stay alive and awake in a vegetative state. However, many people would rather upload their brains to the cloud than take one of these routes. The minimum requirement to keep our consciousness is to maintain a sufficiently healthy and functional brain. In the foreseeable future, this requires a body or at least major organ systems to support the essential metabolism of the brain neurons. Hence, we need the body to live as long as our neurons do to achieve HYL.

Neurons can probably survive a 300-year journey. However, neurogenesis in the brain becomes very slow after birth and neurons are vulnerable to types of damage and degeneration that cause serious consequences. A healthy lifestyle and some dietary supplements can help reduce the chance of neurodegeneration and neuronal death. Still, neurodegeneration and related diseases won't be curable until neuroregeneration and neuroreplacement technologies are mature. This requires more knowledge of neuronal mechanisms and the complex functions of the nervous system. It could take scientists a long time to get there.

If we can eventually control neuronal growth and regeneration, we can artificially increase the number of neurons in the nervous system. As a result, we could have keener senses, thinking, and memory. Since humans rely heavily on the brain, this would be one giant leap for humankind.

The Ultimate Balance

He who lives in harmony with himself lives in harmony with the universe.
—Marcus Aurelius

The brain coordinates the body to regulate the metabolism and functions of different cells. The development of medicine and biotechnology can expand our involvement in these processes to utilize the body for our interest, including reaching and maintaining HYL.

From a cell to a body

Living brings aging. The passing of time carves our bodies. The past is recorded in every growing wrinkle, graying hair, loosening tooth, blurring eye, weakening cell, shortening telomere, and mutating genome.

Aging is more than changes in genes. Studies have demonstrated that aging is also associated with epigenetic changes, which are alterations of gene expression without modifications of gene sequences. For example, RNA interference by ASOs is a common epigenetic process to inhibit protein expression. A series of epigenetic changes are aging-related, such as the remodeling of nucleosomes that is frequently observed in aged cells. In some respects, these aging-related epigenetic changes are like accumulated dust and rust in a car. With high mileage, a car can still be functional, but with all its tear and wear it usually doesn't perform as well as a new car. Aged cells are similar.

Likewise, tissues formed by cells progressively deteriorate in the performance of their functions over time. The same applies to organs formed by tissues, organ systems formed by organs, and the body as a whole. The function of higher anatomical levels depends on the integrated functions of the lower levels. Therefore, to support youth and longevity of the body, we need to maintain health and function at all the lower levels for as long as possible.

An ongoing task

Like in the past millions of years, our battle with the human body will continue in the future. Every day, healthy eating, regular exercise, and a good night's sleep sustain and tune the body. Many medicines and technologies have been developed to help keep the body's balance. For example, painkillers reduce pain and inflammation, ergonomic chairs relax our shoulders and back, artificial kidneys filter blood and remove waste, video games please and enliven the brain. Even advanced surgeries and gene therapies have been developed for the body.

The more we know about the human body, the more things we can do to maintain its balance. For example, sirtuin is a class of proteins that were discovered in the twentieth century. Later, some scientists came to believe that sirtuins are critical for health and longevity. Thus, more and more studies have been conducted on them. Since the activity of some sirtuins depends on nicotinamide adenine dinucleotide (oxidized form: NAD^+), NAD^+ and its precursors have become trendy dietary supplements that claim to boost longevity. Although the true effects of these products are yet to become clear, these studies and commercialization processes reflect the great human desire for health and longevity. Despite the tortuous path, the irresistible power of this desire will continue to push knowledge and technology forward.

The advancement of our knowledge about genes also highlights the beauty and importance of gene delivery as a platform technology. There are so many vital genes in the body that have the potential for artificial manipulation. It will take too long to develop drugs for each one of them, while the current once-in-a-lifetime gene therapy is far from enough to cover all these genes. No one knows when the next longevity gene will be determined or when a true longevity pill will be invented. It would be a pity if a person who seeks health and longevity cannot apply novel discoveries to himself or herself, so that he or she can only wait miserably for aging and death while looking at the happy lives of his or her long-living peers. A fully developed level 3 Miao system can eliminate such problems. With repeated gene delivery, longevity genes that have been identified and will be determined could be artificially activated and adjusted in our bodies. Useful compounds such as NAD^+ could then be synthesized by our cells and for our cells. Since the secrets of living longer and better are found in DNA, we will keep on mining DNA and advancing on this journey even after we can live 300 years.

HYL is a set of sustainable equilibria to maintain the harmony and stability of the body. The ultimate goal is to willingly and actively coordinate metabolism in different parts of the body to reach a long-lasting balance, which is tasks 5 and E in the roadmap (Figure 6). These two tasks are related to all the other tasks, refined and improved. Along with rejuvenation, regeneration, and damage prevention, described in previous chapters, the final task is to maintain the body in HYL or even better states for as long as possible to reach the 300-year or longer goal. The details of such a vast assignment will continuously evolve with our expanding knowledge about the human body.

Different technologies will be used to complement the human brain so as to artificially enhance the desired activities of the body. In an ideal situation, body parameters such as hormone and metabolic levels will be permanently kept around optimal values to maximize the function of different organ systems. Such tasks require the accurate and timely coordination of selected genes in specific groups of cells. Thus, as the diamond drill, a level 3 Miao system will be essential for these tasks. The precise adjustment of DNA by gene delivery will be a powerful addition to current therapies, especially for tasks that are difficult to accomplish by other methods. Eventually, various technologies and methodologies can be consolidated into a systematic approach to harmonizing the body. For example, gene delivery and many medicines function at the molecular level to support the higher levels of the body, while surgeries, transplantations, and other therapies manipulate higher levels to treat the whole body as an organic entity. Timewise, some medicines and first-aid procedures deliver instant effects, while gene delivery and some other medicines operate on the timescale of hours to days. Combining these with other therapies, long-term recovery and improvement of the body may be achieved. Ultimately, all these technologies constitute a comprehensive network to sustain the body beyond its natural limit. As a result, we should be able to live as long as other long-living species.

Omnipotence

Living 300 or more years by guarding our bodies with a group of technologies will be a great achievement for humankind and other lifeforms that are not gifted with a hyper-long lifespan. It will be a huge victory for true rebels who try to escape the reign of the DNA master. If we can willingly adjust our DNA with gene delivery, are we then in total control of our bodies?

Not really. Even with the breakthrough of gene delivery technologies, we won't be close to equalling the might of the brain. A sophisticated level 3 Miao system still has major limitations. The effects of gene delivery rely on the expression or inhibition of genes. If the Miao system is a reagent, it needs to travel through the body to reach the target cells and release the cargo into the cells. The cargo then initiates its mission to express or inhibit genes so as to alter specific cellular pathways. These processes cannot happen in the blink of an eye. It is reasonable to estimate that it may take hours to days to see the effects. This could be too slow for the timely adjusting of many metabolic activities.

Different cell types contain diverse receptors and other structures outside the cell membrane. A gene delivery system can recognize these dissimilarities to specifically target a group of cells. Since receptors and extracellular structures are always shared by more than one cell, it is extremely challenging to accurately identify and target a single cell from the 37 trillion cells in the body. In the foreseeable future, gene delivery systems will also be unable to examine the internal environment of individual cells to determine if the delivery is appropriate. Therefore, gene delivery systems could over-deliver genes to cells of the same kind and lead to unexpected effects.

At any given moment in a typical human cell, thousands of genes are expressed while millions of proteins are working with billions of compounds. Therefore, managing cellular processes needs to be extremely sophisticated. Even with a level 3 Miao system, controlling thousands of genes at the same time seems unachievable, especially given the high speed of metabolism.

A level 3 Miao system will be a game-changing breakthrough in human biotechnology. Still, it won't be comparable with natural cellular regulation networks endorsed by the DNA master. Hence, the roadmap only focuses on key features that can benefit longevity. Our mission is not to make human beings into an almighty lifeform but to reach and keep a sustainable state with expanded lechatelierim.

Let us assume that we have the perfect technology to enable the accurate and timely manipulation of individual genes in specific cells of the body. Moreover, let's imagine that we have a mechanism to precisely identify and manipulate the 37 trillion cells individually. However, even with such powers, we are still far from being omnipotent over the human body.

To systematically control all the cells, we have to accurately determine the internal and external metabolic statuses of individual cells. This is not a simple task. Billions of compounds encounter one another in cells with speeds close to the diffusion-limit, which is greatly faster than most human activities. These compounds are continuously catalyzed by enzymes 10,000 to 1,000,000 times per second. It is extremely difficult to monitor so many exceedingly swift reactions. Moreover, according to Heisenberg's uncertainty principle, the detection of these molecules could be limited at such a microscopic scale. This means we cannot precisely probe all the physical parameters of these small particles.

Let us further assume that we don't need to worry about this basic principle of physics. However, it is still challenging to record the gigantic amount of data generated by countless compounds inside 37 trillion cells. Analyzing and responding to the recorded information is even more difficult. Thus, monitoring and reacting to molecular changes in all cells in the body in a timely fashion doesn't seem plausible. Even the brain cannot regulate everything in every cell. If we want to accurately coordinate all our cells at will, we need to have more power than the DNA master. We need to become Maxwell's demons of our bodies. Hypothetically, we can then smartly utilize metabolism to extend our lifespan indefinitely by sophisticatedly and precisely accomplishing tasks in the roadmap. We will recover and rejuvenate cells to keep the body healthy and young at its different levels for a very long time, just like some of the gods described in ancient mythologies. We will reach the limit of biology. Aging and normal body injuries won't be a problem for us anymore.

However, death still can be triggered by severe damage. True omnipotence can be achieved when we can control all molecules, atoms, subatomic particles, and even elementary particles across the range of our bodies at will. We need to know their statuses and be able to arbitrarily arrange the particles without restraint. In this state, we are reaching, or are even beyond, the power of the universe. Death is no longer a problem since a body can always be reconstituted. Thus, we probably won't be concerned about life and death since they are merely different arrangements of particles. Similarly, a body is not that important as well. As the true Maxwell's demon, the fun thing about existence is probably being able to play with random particles to create all kinds of entities. However, as Heisenberg's uncertainty principle stated, it is impossible to know everything about even a single particle. Therefore, we or even the universe will probably never have such power.

Fortunately, we don't need omnipotence to live 300 or more years.

III. He
(Unity)

We have discussed the roadmap to HYL and the tasks that need to be accomplished. However, living is more than surviving. Let's see what else matters in a 300-year life.

Beyond Human Beings

Those who are able to see beyond the shadows and lies of their culture will never be understood, let alone believed, by the masses.
—Plato

Life expectancy has been continuously increasing for many years. In the Middle Ages, the average life expectancy of English people was only around 30 years. Nowadays, many people live more than twice as long and 30 years is merely the length of time people spend paying back their student loans. More and more people live past 100 years, an age that was considered legendary by our ancestors. Currently, the percentage of centenarians is still less than 1%. However, it is much more probable than many other things in our lives, such as winning the lottery. Moreover, modern science and medicine will continue to make the age of 100 years more reachable.

A 300-year lifespan is over four times longer than what the average person can live today. It has been considered unachievable throughout human history, except in myths and fairy tales. No doubt the goal of reaching the 300-year hallmark will be much harder to achieve than the previous increases in life expectancy. As mentioned in previous chapters, the previous growth of lifespan is within the natural potential of our bodies. Now we are reaching the inherent lifespan boundaries of humankind and it is unlikely that we can naturally live three or four times longer than previous generations. Thus, the real fight for life is about to begin.

If bowhead whales could understand human languages, they would probably wonder why humans worry about aging and dying before hitting the age of 150. "Why don't you eat healthily and keep a healthy lifestyle so that you can live 300 years?" a kind bowhead whale might sincerely ask. "Didn't your mother tell you that?" To them, living 300 years is just repeating the daily routine 109,500 times. However, the human body is not like the body of bowhead whales. Even with special dietary supplements and superior medical care, we know eating healthily and keeping a healthy lifestyle cannot get us to live that long. Thus, making the body capable of living that long by completing tasks in the roadmap is the only way.

This is the path that takes us beyond human beings.

How long is 300 years?

The 300-year goal in this book is based on the estimated lifespan of our neurons. The neurons make us who we are, but we are not yet able to recover or renew functional neurons in our bodies. Therefore, even if we are 300 years old, we likely will still be accompanied by the neurons we were born with. Chances are, we will eventually die because of them. Nevertheless, 300 years is not short and I will be happy with it.

Indeed, 300 years is very long. Although it is only several times longer than a normal person's lifespan, 300 years is quite a chunk when we put it back in history. We are just a little over 2,000 years from 1 CE, which is less than seven 300 years. Three hundred years ago, the world was a very different place. In the eighteenth century, men in England wore stockings and lace cravats while women dressed in fancy gowns. There was no plastic, no T-shirt, no phone, no car, no computer, no air conditioner, no rubber condom, no airplane, no movie, no penicillin, no nuclear bomb, no flush toilet, no credit card, no internet, no satellite, no 9-to-5 job, no constitution, no universal suffrage, no medical insurance, no supermarket, no gas station, not even a hint of modern life.

Many countries, including the United States of America, are less than 300 years old. In the 1720s, the New World was just a scattering of colonies, while countries in the World Island were expanding with blood and iron. The British Empire was becoming the foremost global power while having the Second Hundred Years' War with its neighbor across the Channel. Sweden was stopped by the Great Northern War, leaving the Holy Roman Empire as many fragments of small territories. Peter the Great led the newly formed Russian Empire in the North, while the Ottoman Empire and the Mughal Empire reigned around the Mediterranean Sea and in South Asia. In the Far East, the ascending Great Qing was the new and last imperial dynasty of China. China has the longest continuous written record of history, but it is split into over 20 dynasties. Only two dynasties are longer than 300 years. Most of the time, peace and prosperity are easily crushed by wars and disasters.

We measure world history with our lives.

Some cruel wars in history even lasted over a hundred years, such as the Rebellion of the Five Barbarians in China and the Hundred Years' War between England and France. These wars could be two to three times longer than the average lifespan of those times. Thus, for generations, many people might have thought that fighting and cruelty were quite ordinary. Grandfathers taught grandchildren how to hide and kill since that was how they had been raised. If all that people ever saw in their lives was devastation, it could be difficult for them to preserve virtue and benevolence. In contrast to people who could only live 30 years, a person who could live 100 years during those times might have a different impression of the world. He or she could have the chance to experience harmony in his or her life and so embrace humanity and kindness. Thus, the beauty of peace and love could plant the seed of hope in his or her heart.

Knowing people can freely enjoy their lives is valuable for maintaining the virtues of humankind. A longer lifespan certainly helps for this purpose. Many people who experienced the Cold War are still alive. They may still remember the old days when the world was split by the chilling coldness of the Iron Curtain. For nearly half a century, humankind trembled under the fear of death and destruction. They certainly still remember how love overcame war and globalization brought countries together. People with different skin colors, hair colors, eye colors, backgrounds, cultures, languages, educations, and lifestyles have come from every corner of the world and begun to live happily together to exchange ideas, learn new things, explore one another, create exciting inventions, experience great adventures, and make the world a better place, eye to eye and hand in hand. People with longer lifespans have more opportunities to experience such a beautiful normality for humankind.

Sadly, the wave of globalization is fading again. Over the past few years, wars have arisen, borders have closed, walls have been built, and people have started cursing one another. Nations could easily move against nations and kingdoms against kingdoms. Even in the twenty-first century, many men and women are without food, while the earth shakes in different places. The outbreak of the COVID-19 pandemic has accelerated all these trends. In less than a year, the world has become a different place: people are forced to return home from the global village while rockets with nuclear warheads come out of shadowy caves. Our society may leave a distinct impression on children born after 2019. They may grow up believing that facemasks are a part of common daily dress, schools are computer screens displaying adults' heads, working is parents going upstairs and talking into a phone, foreigners and police officers are bad people... How can we teach children the knowledge of good and evil if all they see is a distorted and abnormal world? No one knows how long this nonsense will last. It may continue for 10, 20, or even more years, but we all know it won't end tomorrow.

The best hope for everyone is to live past the reign of this ruthless virus and the meaningless hostility between nations. People would like to arrive at the harmonious destination called "the ordinary." This is where we shake hands without fear or suspicion. It is where we can directly see one another's smiles. It is where we share our food under the warm bright summer sun, which tans our skins into the same tone. Humans have become more dangerous and offensive throughout our history. However, people have also become more merciful and civilized. We know from our history that ups and downs are common in the stream of time. Things always return to normal eventually, since we are always protected in the lechatelierim of our species.

With a long lifespan, difficult times like the present will be less stressful. If I met a 300-year-old guy at a bar and complained about the current situation, he would probably chuckle and say, "No worries, the Third Plague was much worse... but I still lived through it. I was in London at that time. The whole street shared the same water closet so things got nasty very fast..." If a person knows that he or she will eventually survive through a hard time, that faith will give him or her courage to overcome all difficulties in his or her path. Therefore, a 300-year lifespan will be a powerful weapon against obstacles and challenges in life. It is a mighty placebo that delivers the strongest comfort and support: hope.

So, what will a 300-year-old person see? The rise and fall of empires, the beginnings and finales of wars, the outbreaks and conclusions of pandemics, the emergence of exciting inventions and technologies, the advancements and improvements of human life, and the astonishing epics of humankind from today to the twenty-fourth century. It is difficult to imagine all the stories in the coming years except by experiencing them day by day.

To Green Pastures

Come away, O human child!
To the waters and the wild
With a faery, hand in hand...
—William Butler Yeats, 'The Stolen Child'

We have focused on ourselves, or our bodies more specifically, in the discussions of HYL. However, human beings have never been alone since the birth of our species. People live in clans, groups, families, tribes, societies, and countries. Civilization is built on the exchange of goods and information between individuals. Especially in the modern world, everyone is a member of society, interconnected with others near and far. Therefore, we cannot live 300 years without considering the rest of humankind.

Bread for tomorrow

In today's world, the majority of everyday necessities come from making an exchange with others. Even people who grow their daily food need to obtain all kinds of supplies to sustain their living, such as seeds, fertilizers, and various types of equipment. Of course, a person can choose a primitive lifestyle and separate himself or herself from the rest of the world. However, without industrialized products and professional services, his or her quality of life could be troublesome. Consequently, this person is unlikely to live a long life, as demonstrated by our many ancestors.

The tasks to reach HYL require vast buying powers to obtain products and services from companies and professional agencies. Besides, food, electricity, housing, transportation, and other essentials in daily life need to be purchased from others using currencies. Since exchange with the rest of society

152

is almost inevitable in a 300-year life, personal economy and finance are of great importance. In fact, quite a fortune will be required to reach and keep HYL for three centuries. This needs detailed and sophisticated planning. Starting early is always appreciated, both for finance and health. The earlier a person accumulates enough wealth, the earlier he or she can dedicate it to some of the tasks in the roadmap. As discussed in the telomere chapter, early telomerase gene delivery is likely to double the beneficial effects when compared to the same therapy received at a later age. Moreover, a young body is generally stronger and healthier, which makes rejuvenation easier. Wealth usually grows with age, but a person has to balance this fact with the risk of sickness and death on the path to HYL.

A person with a 300-year lifespan (who will be referred to as *he* for simplicity) has to work or have other means to support living and additional spending during all those years. If the body is periodically rejuvenated, *he* possibly can work throughout a 300-year life. The retirement plan provided by the company *he* has worked for is unlikely to produce enough benefits for over 234 years. Therefore, *he* probably cannot retire at the present retirement age. Instead, *he* may need to work 200 or more years according to current life expectancy and retirement age. Therefore, it is extremely important to plan carefully for career development. A great number of occupations today did not exist 300 years ago. Similarly, many jobs won't exist 300 years from now. Hence, it is unlikely that *he* can keep the same job throughout *his* career. Tenure track professors and medical workers could be the few exceptions. According to a report from the US Bureau of Labor Statistics, many workers spend five years or less in each job. If *he* starts work at 20 and retires at 200, *he* will probably change jobs 36 times during *his* career. Thus, *he* needs to be quick on *his* feet to learn new skills so as to periodically get new jobs.

Risks increase tremendously in the long term and 300 years is not a short time. In such a prolonged period, currencies could be depreciated, devaluated, or even revoked. In the case of countries that have lasted over 300 years, many of them no longer use the same currency as 300 years ago.

The true demon could be inflation. With a 3% average annual inflation rate, $1 will only have a purchasing power of about $0.05 after 100 years. This is a 20-fold depreciation. To match the purchasing power of the current $1, a person needs $19.22 now to fight the depreciation 100 years later. This predicted 20-fold depreciation in 100 years seems too surprising to be true. Unfortunately, the reality is even worse. The Federal Reserve was formed in the USA in 1913 and US inflation has been tracked since then. Ninety-three years later, in 2006, a 20-fold depreciation had already been reached (cumulative inflation: 1,936.4%). An item that cost $1 in 1913 costs $26.29 in 2020 (cumulative inflation: 2,529.1%).

Inflation has been getting worse over the past 50 years. The cumulative inflation from 1913 to 1970 (57 years) was only 291.9%. However, the cumulative inflation from 1970 to 2020 (50 years) was 866.4%. A possible explanation for this acceleration of inflation is the termination of the convertibility of the US dollar to gold in 1971, which ended the Bretton Woods system. After that, currencies around the world no longer worship gold or any other precious metal as the standard of value. Instead, credit money has been widely used to create monetary value through debts. Consequently, gigantic amounts of money have been easily and arbitrarily created, which has greatly accelerated inflation.

Inflation could be deadly over the long term. With a 3% average annual inflation rate, a $1 bill 300 years from now will only have the purchasing power of the current $0.00014. To match the purchasing power of the current $1, a person needs $7,098.51 now to compensate for depreciation over the coming 300 years. This prediction is exceedingly demoralizing. Unfortunately, modern credit money hasn't existed for 300 years yet and it is unclear how this serious problem will be solved. Capitalism will probably require major reforms to survive such a potential catastrophe.

If a person with a 300-year lifespan chooses to retire with *his* savings at 60, *he* will have a hard time fighting inflation over the next 240 years. Even if *he* retires at 200, *his* retirement savings will still depreciate about 20 times in the remaining 100 years. If for some reason *he* cannot maintain a healthy status after the age of 200, the personal care cost will be tremendous for the last 100 years and greatly increase over time. Moreover, periodical economic and financial crises could greatly shrink *his* fortune. Therefore, proper and careful planning will be extremely important for a long lifespan.

Investing seems a reasonable way to fight inflation and improve personal finance for a 300-year life. Compound interest over a long time could be a person's best friend against inflation. With a 5% annual interest, $10,000 will become $22,739,961,286 after 300 years. If a person with a 300-year lifespan has big savings at the beginning, the bank may not be able to afford the interest after several hundred years. Even if *he* only has an average income, *he* has many more years to accumulate savings and propagate wealth through compound interest. With wise investments, *he* should be able to secure a fortune for retirement. Since *he* lives much longer, *he* can afford more waiting time for better investment opportunities. Economic depressions occur about every 10 years, during which people can purchase good assets at bargain prices. For people who can live through six Kondratiev waves (the long economic cycle that lasts about 50 years), waiting for 10 years for good investment opportunities is not a waste of time.

Insurance can be another way to manage financial risks. Many insurance policies utilize compound interest to compensate for inflation. However, insurance companies haven't expected people to live for 300 or more years. Therefore, it is unclear if an insurance policy will still be effective after 200, 300, or 400 years, assuming the insurance company still exists at that time. Nevertheless, the pioneers of human hyper-longevity have to figure out these personal finance problems to support their long lives.

State of my choice

With a 300-year lifespan, a person probably wants to travel around the globe to explore every corner of this beautiful planet. However, *he* still needs to find a dwelling place to rest *his* feet.

When globalization was trendy, the idea of world citizenship was also popular. Its supporters believed that a person's identity should not be limited by geographical and political borders. Yet, globalization is a new concept in the history of humankind. Most of the time, conflicts between countries, cultures, and people have been more common than peace and friendship. Since nations may not last 300 years, a person who can live that long may have to live in different countries during *his* lifetime. National power, government structure, and political beliefs also shift over time. Thus, *he* does not have to choose countries to live in just based on patriotism, ideology, or political systems. In contrast, lifestyle and culture seem more important in the long run. For example, the stability and safety of society, tax rate, cost of living, the quality and accessibility of healthcare systems and education systems, and the taste of food are more critical factors.

Both developed and developing countries could be good choices for living during the many years of *his* life, depending on personal preferences. Although major operations for tasks in the roadmap can be done abroad, regular services should be conducted locally for convenience. Therefore, the countries *he* chooses for *his* 300-year-long life should have enough resources to support these activities. Moreover, state and local laws and regulations should not go against *his* needs.

Red alert

Task 1 in the roadmap (Figure 6) is to avoid danger since deadly external forces are uncontrollable risks. Unintentional injuries caused by accidents are the third leading cause of death in the USA. For young people, homicide is the third leading cause of death, which should be a major concern for rejuvenated people as well.

The importance of safe living cannot be exaggerated. The security of a person's neighborhood and the stability of society should be constantly monitored and prepared in accordance. Since history always repeats itself, people who have experienced a long life should be quite calm about most social disturbances. However, others may get provoked and become irrational. A society in a state of unrest may lose its ability to sufficiently support the tasks in the roadmap. Riots destroy social order and cause many problems. Cultural violence can put everyone in danger, not to mention the possibility of civil wars. These uncertainties are real threats to anyone who would like to live 300 or more years.

People in 2020 know these concerns are not unrealistic. In the case of the USA, Americans have witnessed a divided country, even while facing the menace of a deadly virus. Meanwhile, boosting government debt and depreciation of purchasing power could be an unsolvable problem of modern capitalism. As mentioned previously, inflation could have a tremendous effect within 300 years. It is unclear how the government and economists are going to solve this devastating issue. The economic bubble is like a time bomb that could destroy everything in US society, though the government is still ignoring it, along with soaring debt. Such a situation cannot continue for 300 years. When the economic bubble explodes, the many unemployed, hungry people won't remain peaceful and other social problems are likely to become acute as well. Therefore, anyone who wants to live 300 years needs to prepare before the time comes.

Civil wars are the most intense conflicts to occur within the same country. They can last a long time, leading to a large number of casualties and the destruction of significant resources. In the American Civil War, about 3% of the population lost their lives. Civil wars in other countries have been even more destructive. For example, with its long history, China has had numerous civil wars that in total lasted more than a thousand years. A number of them resulted in over 10 million casualties. For example, the battle between the Three Kingdoms (220–280 CE) killed about 90% of the population of that time. Probably the best way to avoid such tragic events is to escape before the situation worsens.

Almost every day, there are wars happening somewhere on Earth between countries. Consequently, so many people lose their lives while defending their homelands. For example, both the Soviet Union and China had over 20 million casualties in World War II. Since most of the wars in history happened in Eurasia, North America seems a comparably safer place. Besides, with the military power of the United States, invasions are unlikely to happen inside its borders. Still, a person living in the USA might get enlisted for overseas military operations, though rejuvenated people are probably too old, officially, to serve. Moreover, nuclear weapons threaten all human beings. With thousands of warheads on duty around the world, it will be impossible to survive if the coming nuclear warfare causes the extinction of humankind.

Humankind vs. Wild

Choose only one master — nature.
— Rembrandt van Rijn

Nature cannot sustain itself if all humans live 300 years. Nowadays, there are around 8 billion people globally, who live 72 years on average. See how many problems we have already created: global warming, serious pollution, extinction of species, hydric stress, and many more. Human beings are using more resources than Earth can afford and have caused more damage to the environment in the past 100 years than in the earlier 1 billion years combined. An average American annually uses nearly 90,000 kilowatt-hours of energy, which is about the energy of 2,500 gallons of gasoline. Each American also consumes about 1 ton of food each year, which is heavier than 1,300 chickens. Such a huge resource consumption has never been seen before in Earth's history. Many scientists believe that human activities in the past 50 years have surpassed Earth's renewability. Earth Overshoot Day is the date each year when human consumption exceeds what nature can regenerate. It was 29 December in 1970 and became 29 July in 2019. Technically speaking, humans need about 1.7 Earths to support our current lifestyle. Even if we stopped squandering the ecosystem today, it could take Earth millions of years to recover. It is difficult to predict if humankind can survive the next 300 years by continuing what we are doing. However, we will probably become extinct soon if everyone has a 300-year life expectancy.

Currently, a generation is about 25 years, which is the time required for a child to grow up and have children. With a 72-year life expectancy, a family generally has 3 to 4 generations of people. If everyone has a 300-year life expectancy, a family could have 12 generations of people. This means tripling or quadrupling the current world population. Moreover, since people will be rejuvenated, mating and birthing processes will no longer be stopped by aging. Therefore, a person's new baby could have the same age as his or her great-great-great-great-great-great-great-great-grandchildren. Consequently, the world population could rocket sky-high. To maintain the same lifestyle, humans may need ten or more Earths for consumption. It will be a tragedy for all species on this planet. Before interstellar travel and extraterrestrial colonies are feasible, we or later generations will probably have to pay the price eventually and get harshly punished by Mother Nature.

Involution

Human society may also not be able to sustain itself if all of us have a 300-year life expectancy. With many times more population, social problems could dramatically worsen. Resources will become much more limited and social inequality could increase to a dangerous level. Since people can work for over 200 years, retirement will be greatly postponed. As a result, opportunities for young people will dramatically shrink and the unemployment rate will escalate. People may have to spend decades on education and pay back their student loans in a hundred years or more. Thus, social class solidification could intensify and economic growth could be disrupted. Consequently, the middle class will shrink and more poor people will require assistance from the government. However, government efficiency will likely decrease due to the significantly increased population, while more debt has to be raised to support its daily functions. Medical systems could also become shaky due to the huge population burden. Even with industrial agriculture, it would be difficult to feed so many people. Many species will forever lose their habitats to farmlands or be eaten to extinction. Many people will struggle with starvation and work like slaves throughout their long lives.

No matter how dedicated they are, saving money will still be difficult due to the devastating effect of inflation in the long run and the inevitable salary decrease caused by overpopulation.

With over ten generations living at the same time, families could become gigantic, while current family relationships may no longer exist. Even remembering all the names of family members and feeding so many mouths will not be easy tasks. The government may have to establish birth-planning programs to save humankind and Earth. Such policies will certainly provoke various religious, ethnic, and social groups.

Due to growing social issues, conflicts in a divided society could become more intense. Historic overpopulations in Eurasia usually led to revolt and war. Ancient societies were always rebalanced after physically removing a large percentage of the population, so the land was enough to support the survivors. With modern weaponry and a great number of armed people, the consequences of social conflicts could be nasty as hell. This does not sound like an ideal future.

What if Earth can provide enough resources even if overpopulated by human beings?

Dr. John B. Calhoun conducted a series of interesting ethological experiments in the 1960s. In one of them, he created a mouse universe that would be able to hold around 4,000 mice with an unlimited supply of food yet no predators. Eight mice were introduced into the mouse universe. In less than a year, the population had increased over 80 times. However, the growth then slowed down and the community started to break down, accompanied by unusual actions such as the harming of young mice by older mice. In the second year, the mouse community experienced their last surviving birth and peaked, with a population that was only 60% of the designed capacity of the mouse universe. Later, the population declined and less than 30 mice survived in the fourth year. The survivors didn't mate even after they were moved to other places. Eventually, the entire population was extinct.

Although humans and mice behave differently and have distinct social structures, this experiment still metaphorically described a potential ending of an overpopulated society. The twisted "behavioral sink" caused by overcrowding is always a threat to humankind, no matter if our life expectancy is 72 years or 300 years.

The Proud Few

Denn das allein
Unterscheidet ihn
Von allen Wesen
(For that alone
Makes him distinct
From every other being)
—Johann von Goethe, 'Das Göttliche'

If Earth is still our only dwelling place, human beings cannot afford to have a universal 300-year life expectancy. Even if technology is no longer a problem, both natural and social issues will prevent it from happening. Therefore, if HYL is achievable, it won't be available to everyone. This could lead to the greatest social disaster ever.

"All men are created equal"

The founders of the United States wrote down this great and touching statement as the foundation of that nation. However, the definitions of "all," "men," "created," and "equal" have been argued over and fought for since their day. This beautiful belief is difficult to achieve in practice since everyone wants a better life. What determines whether a person, but not his or her peers, deserves a better education, more money, greater power, or a bigger house? A person's inspiration and perspiration could be one answer—a politically correct one.

However, societies, like Mother Nature, have never been truly fair towards talent and hard work. Opportunities are always twisted by skin color, gender, looks, family background, ideology, politics, bribery, and many other things. If all men *and women and other human beings* are created equal, then equality probably only means that we all have a human body.

Unfortunately, even this frank equality is artificially divided into different classes and sealed with stereotypes. In real life, social balance is always politically incorrectly tilted towards people who have advantages. In modern capitalism, common advantages come in the forms of more money, more power, and more social connections. The concentration of social advantages is a spontaneous chain reaction that leads to the widening of social inequality in the world. In the USA nowadays, the top 1% of the population is 15 times wealthier than the bottom 50% combined. Thus, even if men *and women and other human beings* are created equal, they for sure don't live equally.

If people are born unequally and live with inequality throughout their lives, it is unlikely that the opportunity to live longer will be evenly distributed to everyone. According to the renewability of Earth, it may only be able to afford a situation where less than 1%, or even less than 0.001%, of the population enjoy a 300-year lifespan. The richest 1% or 0.001% of people will likely be the first group to benefit from a much longer life. Throughout their multi-century-long life, fortune and power will continuously accumulate in their hands. In contrast, the general public will work tirelessly for food like humanized tools. Consequently, the already massive wealth inequality could skyrocket. Eventually, the difference in lifetime earnings of 300-year-olds and normal people will become much larger than that between ancient slave owners and slaves. Thus, 300-year-olds could become extremely wealthy and powerful.

In honey bee society, queens live for 3–4 years while worker bees live only for weeks. Along with the difference in social power between queens and worker bees, such a huge inequality in lifespan contributes to the establishment of the eusociality of bee communities. Similarly, a much longer lifespan could become the unique biological distinction of a tiny percentage of very powerful people. This could ultimately reshape human society.

So far, death is the only thing that is truly equal for all human beings. With or without fancy medication and meticulous care, everyone gets sick, feels pain, and faces death's scythe within a *reasonably comparable* life expectancy. However, the *few* who can live much longer will break this sole equality. They can happily plan for the coming 200 and more years while most people age, suffer, and die. The provoked rage of the general public will be furious. Especially if the *few* are also the richest and most powerful people in the world, they will be hated more than anyone in history.

When the *few* look at the general public, they may feel pride in their own superiority. With the stimulation of wealth and power, this pride could escalate to arrogance. They may feel like Brahmins in the Indian caste system and treat others like Shudras. However, for modern people who already have freedom and equality rooted in their minds, it won't be easy to establish an official slavery system. Instead, the *few* may hide from the public to avoid disclosing their long and prosperous lives. Alternatively, they may show their charm and kindness in public to ease the hostility, for example by offering members of the general public limited opportunities to join them. The rich and powerful have been doing similar things for a long time, but a great lifespan boost will make the situation more complicated. Since 300-year-olds will always be the minority, potential conflicts with the rest of the population will remain an unsolvable problem.

Although genetically almost identical, the *few* are no doubt quite distinct from normal *Homo sapiens*. The *few* could even be treated as a different species or a subspecies in some respects. Therefore, racial discrimination is highly possible. The discrimination could be unidirectional or bidirectional, but either way, it can split societies and result in conflicts.

However, there is no doubt that many people will want to be a member of the *few*.

The lightning comes

Lifespan extension won't be a universal charity and seats to join the *few* are limited. Thus, if a technology or a product is able to extend the human lifespan to 300 years, it won't be advertised in the newspapers. Hence, how to find out if such a technology has been developed?

The fundamental requirement of the roadmap to HYL is a *reliable* gene delivery system. It has to be able to repeatedly deliver genes to the human body, efficiently and without toxicity or other adverse effects. The development of such a system determines how soon we can start marching on our path to HYL. Currently, there are many gene delivery technologies available. Some of them have been commercialized while others are still under development. Most of these technologies have apparent defects so that it is difficult to predict which technology will become the first Miao system. As previously described, the development of a Miao system may have different stages. Thus, even a dull level 0 system that has not been clinically used has the potential of becoming the future savior. Scientists who study gene delivery and read this book may realize the importance of their work for the future of humankind. If they decide to conceal their findings, it would be nearly impossible for others to know that such technology already exists.

Besides a reliable gene delivery system, some other technologies are also essential for accomplishing the roadmap, such as tissue regeneration. Studies on the molecular mechanisms of longevity-related genes and associated drug developments are important as well. However, no one knows exactly when such technologies will be developed. Before the big leap forward comes, we have to wait for it patiently.

The Silent Observer

It takes a long time to become young.
—Pablo Picasso

If one person or a few lucky persons (still referred to as *he* for simplicity) successfully developed a technology to enable a 300-year lifespan, what would *his* options be? In this chapter, we will brainstorm such a scenario. These plots are purely fictitious and any similarity to real life is just coincidental.

Blue pill and red pill

After all the excitement has faded away, *he* needs to decide what to do with *his* technology.

He can announce it publicly, hoping everyone will benefit from the invention. However, unless *he* is already a renowned scientist, the reception won't be very enthusiastic. Most people won't notice this breakthrough. Even if they do, chances are the majority won't care about it or believe it at all. This is simple to understand: people don't expect such technologies to work and there have been so many failed cases in history. Some people will laugh at *him* while some may call *him* a liar. The believers and nosy journalists will try to dig out everything about *him*. Extremists may discriminate against *him*, hate *him*, or even attack *him* for whatever reason. Meanwhile, the government and other researchers will want *his* secrets. Even if *he* chooses to tell them everything, it will take quite a long time for them to believe. Similarly, if *he* tells them something wrong, it may take a long time for them to find out and they will likely get very angry. If *he* chooses not to disclose the details, they may think *he* is a liar and therefore *his* reputation is at risk. Alternatively, they may try to figure *his* technology out by forcefully inspecting *his* data or even taking specimens from *his* body.

If people finally believe *him*, *he* will instantly become the hero of the world. If not, *he* has enough life ahead of *him* to wait for that day to come. However, with great fame comes great risk. It is expected that every country in the world will want *him*, while the country *he* is in will do everything to keep *him*. There could be conflicts or even wars. Consequently, *he* may not be able to travel abroad anymore. Even in *his* own country, *he* will be heavily protected and partially lose *his* freedom. In this case, people who work with *him* may become the core members of the *few*. Eventually, the world may treat *him* as a hero or a demon, or both.

Instead, *he* can privately disclose *his* technology to the government without notifying the general public. The absence of public awareness may protect *him* from being harassed by outsiders. However, there could be other risks. For example, if *he* reports directly to *his* immediate manager, the manager may steal *his* invention. The manager may reveal it to the public and take all the fame and risks. Moreover, *his* life could be in danger if the government decided to cover up the secret. Without public supervision, things could easily get nasty. In those situations, *he* may have to flee to other countries or publicize the secrets for *his* safety. However, if *he* gets attention and support directly from the upper echelons of the government, *he* may receive unlimited resources to perfect *his* technology. Consequently, those people from the government are likely to form the central hub of the *few* with *him*. It will then become challenging to balance the focus of such a diverse team, especially if the powerful people involved have distinct interests. Eventually, *he* may lose control of *his* technology and disappear in the stream of history.

If *he* needs an ally, *he* can talk with *his* friends about the new technology. However, they have to be able to keep *his* secret. Chances are, *his* friends also want to live longer. Thus, more people get an extended lifespan if they can make it into his close circle. This could be the origin of the *few*. However, *his* friends may have their friends and families who want to live longer as well. Consequently, the squad could soon become a clan. If this process continues, even if they don't intend to let it happen, the technology will eventually be exposed to the public.

If *he* would like a quiet and "normal" life, *he* could keep the secret within *his* family or even just to *himself*. If so, we the general public won't find a hint about the technology anywhere. Someone else may eventually develop something similar, but *he* could probably hide it for many years.

Living in countries with low population density will likely help keep *his* secret since *his* young appearance will draw less attention. In the long run, *he* still needs to prepare to move to other places, fake *his* death, or change *his* identity completely. People around *him* may become suspicious when *he* is 50 or 60 years old but still looks young. The suspicion will increase greatly when *he* reaches the age of 70 or 80 years. At this point, *he* probably has to move to another place and live with a forged juvenile identity: it is unusual for someone with a young appearance to claim that he is an older person, and *he* may attract news crews to *his* home. However, if *he* changes *his* identity, *he* may lose the opportunity to prove *himself* later. By that time, many of *his* old friends have probably already passed away. Even if they are still alive, they are not likely to remember or be able to recognize *him* anymore. Anyway, if *he* lives carefully, people around *him* may not realize any abnormality. Many countries keep a record of centenarians and even 90-year-olds for elderly care and *he* will draw attention from the government without a new identity. When *he* is 110 or 120 years old, *he* could become the oldest living person in that country or even in the whole world. At that time, if *he* hasn't changed his identity, it will be quite difficult for *him* to explain *his* young appearance. *He* could disguise himself with a more "senior" appearance, but it wouldn't pass any physical examination. Consequently, *he* could be misrecognized as *his* grandson who is trying to steal *his* retirement benefits and it could be troublesome.

He could choose to announce *his* real identity at that time and the world will be shocked with amazement. If *he* doesn't uncover the secret of *his* technology, some people may think *he* is a religious miracle, while others may think *he* is a mutant that is a danger to humankind. Scientists will become extremely curious about *his* body and thorough examinations will be inevitable. If the signs of genetic modifications in *his* genome are obvious, *his* secret will be easily exposed by a simple blood or DNA sample. However, if *he* only uses transient gene delivery, *his* secret can remain a mystery. This may not be a good thing. Scientists may want more and bigger parts of *his* body for testing, which may not be pleasant. If *he* lives in an autocratic country, *he* may be forced to accept these examinations.

The general public may also have unrealistic fantasies about *his* body. Some women may want to have a baby with *him*. It is unclear if the rejuvenated body will be vigorous enough for such burdens. Other people may have other ideas, some of which may not be pleasant. In the famous ancient Chinese novel *Xi You Ji* (Journey to the West), the Monkey King, Sun Wukong, protected the Chinese monk Tang Sanzang from attacks of all kinds coming from the *Yao Guai* (bewitched monsters) throughout their journey across Asia. The reason that so many *Yao Guai* attacked Tang Sanzang is that they believed they would become immortal if they ate Tang Sanzang's flesh, which would taste even better if cooked by steaming. This could be the worst situation for a person who has a 300-year lifespan.

Nevertheless, it would be difficult to keep *his* secret for 300 years and *he* has to be able to sustain *his* livelihood for that length of time. *He* could choose to publicly disclose *his* technology when *he* is at a great age (probably over 120). The effects of *his* technology will be very convincing at that time and *he* will instantly become a national treasure.

If *he* figures out a way to keep *his* secret during *his* hyperlong life, *he* can spend *his* time peacefully in a quiet corner somewhere on Earth, living as a silent observer of humankind. *He* can live through the growth and decline of great nations, experience the good and bad of human society, witness wars and pandemics, watch fancy inventions reshaping daily life, even see the first colony on another planet... If *he* records *his* observations and thoughts along the way, that would be an interesting book to read.

Waste time wisely

With a much longer lifespan, the silent observer should have more time to spend on different things. Hopefully, the extended life won't all be used just for making money. Family time is precious, though staying with family members for centuries could be stressful for some people. Anyway, *he* will encounter many more people in *his* lifetime to create more exciting stories. Designing and building *his* own house and garden could be a great plan. There will be enough time to master all the handyman skills and gradually extend the landscaping for the perfect home. Traveling around the world and experiencing different cultures would be fascinating and could take many years. *He* has plenty of time to develop new hobbies, practice new skills, and learn new things. *He* can also immerse *himself* in various sports and arts, and build new friendships along the way. Three hundred years is long enough to obtain multiple advanced degrees to master a series of professions, and thus to experience different aspects of human civilization. Reading is also an engaging pastime and *he* can enjoy immersing *himself* freely in the ocean of masterpieces for centuries. There are just so many things to experience that *he* will never feel *he* has had enough.

Despite all the troubles that come with a hyper-long life, a 300-year HYL will be a thrilling adventure. Encountering the world with an always healthy and young body for hundreds of years is like reliving many lives, but always fresh, knowledgeable, adventurous, experienced, and full of enthusiasm and excitement. Even thinking about the opportunities that a hyper-long life brings can energize a person's tiring heart to hope for a new start. Life is good and time is cool.

Inevitable Death

We die only once, and for such a long time.
—Molière

Long-living organisms all die eventually. After living for hundreds or thousands of years, their bodies finally are sufficiently worn and lead them to rest in peace. After staying in HYL for 300 or more years, we also have to face the same destiny. If all our cells, including neurons, can be repeatedly regenerated and efficiently replaced, we can probably live indefinitely. It is unclear for how long such a body can survive, or how it will die.

Nevertheless, even if a body can function properly for thousands of years, it will still die eventually. Maybe future generations will be able to keep the body or the consciousness alive for millions of years, which is beyond the timescale that we can reasonably imagine. This could be done by extensively remodeling the body or uploading the mind to a stronghold. However, even if we can live for that long, we are still unlikely to outlive Earth. Ultimately, even if we can escape to other planets or drift in space, the universe also has its ending.

If we enjoyed a 300-year life, could we magnanimously face the final moment and graciously accept it? Would we be spoiled by the extra years and have even more desire for life? Would we have more fear of death than when we were 30?

Only time can tell.

No matter for how long we try to postpone it, we have to face the ultimate and final question someday. The answer may hide in the hope of reincarnation. The answer may shine in the grace of the religious afterlife. The answer may dwell in an ancient family tradition. The answer may exist in the deepest ego of free will. The answer may reside in scientific analyses and deductive logic. The answer may lie in the serenity of philosophical speculation. The answer may have sneaked inside a niche of animal instinct. The answer may already be known by the DNA master and the universe.

The answer is there.

IV. Yi
(Oneness)

Now we know what we may face in a hyper-long life, we will discuss a few topics beyond the scope of a normal 300-year HYL.

Forward to the Future

It has become appallingly obvious that our technology has exceeded our humanity.
—Albert Einstein

A mature gene delivery system will bring dramatic changes to every aspect of human life. Completing tasks in the roadmap for a 300-year life is only one of its many applications.

More than *Homo sapiens*

A sophisticated Miao system can accurately regulate our genes, which could have many interesting and powerful functions. In the roadmap, one of its applications is to guide the release of different hormones to artificially coordinate the balance and rhythms of our metabolism. Likewise, it can be used to further boost the potentials of the human body by adjusting hormone levels. For example, in certain circumstances, a person can use a controlled release of epinephrine to enhance his or her memory or physical abilities. He or she can also use the manual release of dopamine to keep positivity and prevent depression. Moreover, we mentioned that gene delivery may help to balance insulin levels for people with diabetes. Similarly, it can be used to regulate leptin levels for weight management. Of course, the hormone levels in these examples need to be carefully monitored and accurately adjusted.

Continuously regulating hormone levels can also induce long-term effects, which could be particularly beneficial for certain specialists such as professional athletes. Some performance-enhancing hormones are naturally synthesized by the human body. Their levels can be increased to improve athletic performance and it may not be recognized as doping. Nevertheless, the Olympic committee won't like it. However, they will have a hard time banning or even detecting performance enhancement induced by hormone gene delivery. For example, hormone levels can be adjusted by gene delivery in a timely fashion to pass doping tests. Moreover, gene delivery can provoke the synthesis of specific enzymes to break down hormones and other drugs in urine to avoid detection. Besides athletes, artificial hormone adjustment may also be beneficial for people who work long hours or need extra concentration. Gene delivery can improve their performance and reduce the burdens on their bodies. If gene delivery is adequately affordable, convenient, and effective, everyone can use it for his or her work. Brain-workers can enhance their focus and thinking skills, while manual workers can have improved strength and endurance. Society will then become more efficient with boosted productivity.

Gene delivery can command our cells to synthesize specific compounds and proteins for our purposes. For example, all vitamins could be synthesized in our bodies so that we no longer need to worry about vitamin deficiency. As a result, intake of vitamins from foods isn't vital anymore. Other than adjusting hormones to stimulate muscle growth, we can deliver genes to directly induce muscle cell proliferation and make more myofibrillar proteins to enhance muscular strength. This could be ideal for bodybuilders, since taking steroids and bearing the adverse effects are not needed. Likewise, bone density can be enhanced, which could be helpful for martial artists and other athletes. We can also produce more opsins in the eyes to improve vision, especially night vision. Similar enhancements can be applied to other senses such as hearing and smell by increasing the number of sensory receptors or optimizing the function of sensory neurons. These modifications certainly need careful examination and correction. We can even replace human proteins with better or more functional homologs from other species to have better senses. If we can see ultraviolet like cats and hear ultrasound like bats, we will experience the world in a whole new way.

Adjusting proteins in our bodies can also bring better experiences to our daily life. For example, alcohol dehydrogenase detoxifies the ethanol we drink. If we have more of this enzyme in the liver, we can have more shots than ever before. Moreover, we can utilize other proteins to suppress ROS and relieve DNA damage after we drink. Another example is amylase, which breaks down starch to produce glucose. Increasing the amount of amylase in our mouth may improve digestion and enhance the sweetness in every bite we take. Similarly, pepsin and lactase digest protein and lactose in the stomach and small intestine, the increment of which may enhance absorption and reduce food intolerance.

Gene delivery can also be used to change our looks. For example, we can control the synthesis of melanin in our skin to adjust skin color. Without going to the beach, we can tan our skin at home. Similarly, we may change the color of our hair and lips without makeup. Even fancier, we can induce the production of different pigments to introduce novel colors to our skin and hair. For example, psittacofulvin and turacoverdin from birds have vivid red and green colors that have not been seen in the human body. Eye colors may be similarly changed. Furthermore, some proteins glow in the dark, so these can be made into fancy tattoos. Using transient gene delivery, these tattoos are not permanent and people can switch between different styles as they wish. Besides skin color, we can use gene delivery to alter our height, body type, and hair volume. Ultimately, a person can guide the growth of skin and bones to arbitrarily change his or her appearance at will.

Furthermore, we can express nonhuman genes in our bodies to gain novel abilities. For example, antifreeze proteins and thermostable proteins from some organisms enable them to survive in extreme environments. If these proteins are expressed in the human body, people could have enhanced cold or hot resistance, which may support the body for cryonics. Since humans do not express cellulase in the digestive system, we cannot break down cellulose and get energy from it. If we express cellulase in our bodies, we can then eat plants like herbivores. Combined with enzymes that produce essential amino acids and vitamins, vegetarians and vegans can completely rely on plant-based foods to live. These modifications could also help solve the global food problem.

Plants, algae, and bacteria have many photosynthesis proteins, which store energy directly from sunlight. If we integrate them into our skin, we may need less food to survive. However, these photosynthetic systems require the coordination of multiple complicated proteins and even isolated organelles, which could be extremely challenging to implement artificially.

With a reliable gene delivery system, everyone's body could become a biochemical factory. We can use it to synthesize numerous kinds of proteins and compounds. An advantage of the human body is that it generates protein post-translational modifications that are unique to humans. Therefore, proteins synthesized by our bodies are most suitable for our usage and consumption. In the future, people may lease their bodies to synthesize antibodies or other functional proteins for pharmaceutical and biotechnology companies. The products are manufactured in the body after gene delivery and collected from blood or secretions. This could be a passive income stream that everyone can have.

The perfect kid

There are so many functions we would like to implement into our bodies to improve our lives. However, even with a level 3

Miao system, it could be remarkably difficult to deliver all the genes. Therefore, it may not be plausible to append so many modifications to the body. A much easier and more reliable strategy is to create the perfect human from a fertilized human zygote or embryo.

This approach has major safety and ethical concerns. In 2018, Chinese researchers conducted the world's first genome-editing experiment on human embryos and resulted in genetically modified human children. They aimed to gain resistance to HIV. However, the CRISPR/Cas9 system they used has a high off-target error rate. As a result, the unfortunate genome-edited babies did not gain resistance to HIV. Instead, they received off-target modifications that may impact essential functions of their bodies, which sadly will accompany them throughout their lives and even be passed to their descendants. Such an irresponsible experiment is a disgrace for science and all human beings. Safety should always be the top priority of embryotic genome editing with no excuses. If technologies cannot guarantee a safe and accurate result, such experiments should never be conducted. Moreover, genetically modified human zygotes and embryos can cause endless ethical problems.

Once technologies are safe and reliable, it is predictable that someone will eventually conduct a similar experiment. If it fails, the country's government will publicly condemn the researcher, just as the Chinese government did previously. If it succeeds, the country's government will likely support the researcher, at least secretly. The reason is simple: such technology can bring enormous benefits to a country. Every government wants its citizens to be superhumans, just like all parents want their kids to be healthy, strong, and smart. Utilizing human-guided evolution by genome editing to only select the beneficial traits for "producing" perfect kids is the ultimate solution to fulfill such an expectation. This approach is much more powerful, efficient, and comprehensive than any good, bad, and ugly eugenic attempts in history. Although many traits are also influenced by environmental factors, advantageous genes continuously deliver positive effects before and after birth. Moreover, repeated gene deliveries can be used to guide development throughout the lifetimes of these perfect kids. Chances are, before long, the country will have numerous smarter, stronger, and healthier citizens growing up from perfect kids. This country then is likely to have greater average productivity than any other country and could become a leading power in the world shortly after. No government can resist the opportunity to have such a future.

Genetically modified human zygotes or embryos may first be utilized by desperate parents who have serious inherited diseases and then gradually spread through the population. For example, the Chinese couple who allowed researchers to conduct the world's first genome-editing experiment on their children are HIV carriers. Once the procedure is fully developed, future parents will likely become fanatic about getting the "best" traits for their children-to-be. Engineered children could thus be biologically distinct from their parents, which would alter the natural path of evolution created by the DNA master. After several generations, as the work of our own hands, humans may no longer be humans.

Even with suitable technologies, making a perfect kid is still not straightforward. Many traits are contributed by a series of genetic factors, whose relations are yet to be determined. Moreover, many traits don't even have an optimal solution. For example, there isn't a universally best height. Although extreme heights could be pathogenic, regular heights don't have major health concerns and are diverse enough for human variability. Being either tall or short is preferred by some people and suitable for a wide range of professions. Similarly, appearance also varies dramatically and so is a matter of aesthetics. If parents can choose the way their children look, the world will be filled with beautiful guys and gals that resemble Hollywood stars and supermodels.

The traits people like may not always be good. For example, enhanced intelligence will be one of the first characteristics that parents want for their babies through genetic engineering. However, filling the world with smart people could be a bad thing. Society could become super dull and boring if everyone is a bright, rational, logical, calculating, and self-interested *Homo economicus* as portrayed by economists. Since resources in a society are always limited, social competition will become fierce when people all have the same set of smart genes. Similarly, zero-sum games between countries could turn out even more risky and dangerous with more cool and scheming minds calculating behind the scenes. At least one thing is known for sure: not all jobs are suitable for smart people and the best decisions in history are not always made by the brightest brains.

Adding new functions to human zygotes or embryos through genome editing could be highly risky. It is hard to predict all the adverse effects since problems may show up many years after. In comparison, gene delivery in adults is much more manageable. Trial-and-error is expected when making perfect kids, but this could become a huge burden for the parents. Therefore, although raising perfect kids could bring a great advantage to a country, failures could be catastrophic as well. Nevertheless, the reliability of technologies and a comprehensive understanding of related molecular mechanisms are the absolute prerequisites. Toxic gene delivery systems and error-prone genome editing systems should never be tolerated.

The universe my destination

Scientific research and technological development never cease. Many advancements could happen in 300 years. Thus, the more years we have, the more opportunities we will get to extend our lives with novel technologies.

An intriguing breakthrough could happen in nanorobotics, which creates controllable devices of various sizes in the micrometer to millimeter range. Such machines are still in a stage of primitive development, but they could have great potential once completed. These robots are small enough to travel inside blood vessels or even dive into cells. They can have numerous applications, such as monitoring metabolism, delivering small cargos and drugs, cleaning blood vessels, and so on. These nanorobots can complement gene delivery systems to make body maintenance much easier. For example, blood vessel bypass or transplant may not be required if clots can be safely and efficiently removed. However, such tasks are not simple, so the robots need to be precisely controlled manually or through sophisticated software. Moreover, it would be great if they are made of biodegradable materials that can be recycled by human metabolism to minimize potential malfunctions.

Stem cell technology and organ regeneration are also attractive fields. As mentioned in previous chapters, they can repair tissue and organ damage to keep the body new. Transplantation of organs or even organ systems may still be needed in HYL and reliable donor sources are always in demand. Organs grown in flasks or from genetically modified animals could be the ultimate solution. Moreover, the technical and ethical issues associated with manipulating human zygotes and embryos may be solved in the future. Afterward, human clones could become common and alter our society.

In the long run, developments in neuroscience could probably lead to reliable neuroregeneration. Consequently, the expiration date of the brain could be largely extended. As discussed earlier, transferring the brain to a new body to get young again sounds like a fascinating strategy. If brain exchange or mind transfer is eventually feasible, we may no longer need to care about our bodies as much as described in this book. If possible, mind uploading is an option to escape from the restrictions of the flesh once and for all and to live happily ever after in binary signals. These technologies are controversial and challenging to develop. However, they may ultimately reshape human beings in the future.

The advancement of technologies may lead humankind out of our home planet. If we live in space or colonize other planets, we will need to adapt to distinct environments and gravities. For this purpose, certain modifications of the body may be required and a Miao system will be helpful for this mission. Such human-induced evolution may finally differentiate people on Earth, in space, and on other planets. Meanwhile, hypothetically, all human jobs could ultimately be performed by computers and robots, while people just physically or virtually enjoy their lives.

So many things are possible with more time.

Every Person Must Play a Part

Time is a drug. Too much of it kills you.
—Sir Terence Pratchett, 'Small Gods'

In this chapter, we will continue to brainstorm the scenario of one or a few lucky persons (still referred to as *he*) who have developed a technology to enable a 300-year lifespan. These plots are still purely fictitious and any similarity to real life is just coincidental.

A grand opening

As mentioned previously, a functional Miao system has numerous applications besides helping people reach HYL. Since many people will want *his* technology, *he* may need to patent it if *he* chooses to publicize *his* invention. However, a patent doesn't mean anything if it cannot be defended in court. This could be very expensive: in the USA, the average litigation cost of a patent infringement case is approximately $4 million now. Some big companies blatantly infringe the patents of startups since they cannot afford to sue. *He* needs to find ways and money to defend *his* patents. Otherwise, *his* invention will be spread around the world by others. Yet, for technology that is so important, others will try to put their hands on it no matter what action *he* takes. Moreover, a patent is not forever. Its term is usually 20 years, which is much shorter than 300 years. *He* may extend the protection by filing new patents, but *his* technology will be shared with the rest of the world eventually. Hence, *he* may need to think about the consequences of the widespread use of *his* technology beforehand.

If *his* technology is only semifinished, *he* could announce *his* discovery and incorporate around the technology to continue research and development in a company. Thus, *he* probably needs to pitch to investors to raise money. Investors care more about the return of their investment and this may not align with the advancement of *his* invention. Since the development of biotechnologies can take a long time, it doesn't meet the expectation of many investors because long-term risks are difficult to manage. *He* could try to persuade investors with *his* goal to extend life to 300 or more years (and maybe use this book as one of *his* references). However, investors will probably be more prone to spend money on a company that is doing identical things to the other 50 companies in a trendy field. Even if *he* gets investment for *his* startup, *he* has to put up with unfair terms and continuous pressure from investors. Chances are, *he* will eventually lose control of the company and *his* aim of increasing lifespan with *his* technology will be completely distorted by novices who are then in charge. Insightful investors are always difficult to find and even harder to convince. Christopher Columbus spent over 10 years meeting with various kings and queens around Europe before Isabella I of Castile finally agreed to sponsor the voyages to America. If *he* is fortunate enough, *he* can get support from investors who share the same vision with *him* on *his* technology.

However, nobody knows if the technology will work or not and it may take years to find out. They can work quietly until the technology is fully developed. Although this rarely happens, if the investors' goal is only a hyper-long life and not money, they don't need to reveal their findings at all. They may secretly become the founders of the *few*. Alternatively, they can publicly announce at the beginning that the company is aiming at reaching a 300-year lifespan. They would certainly get some news coverage, though no one would expect it to work. Therefore, if the technology fails or they hide their success in the future, the general public won't pay much attention to it. In contrast, if they decide to broadcast their accomplishment when the technology is mature, the public won't be too surprised since the news was reported before. This could make selling their products easier if they choose to commercialize the technology. Nevertheless, the business world is harsh, unforgiving, and more intertwined with other interests than scientific research. *He* could earn a lot of fame and fortune, but it may not always be a blessing.

Even if a person knows that the technology doesn't work, he or she can exaggerate its ability and sell products. Chances are, this person will still make a lot of money and enjoy a happy life. This doesn't seem a bad plan for someone with a normal lifespan. One of the beauties of longevity products is that there are always believers and it takes a whole lifetime to figure out the outcome.

Sheng Si Bu

In Chinese mythology, death is governed by the office of Yan Luo Wang (the king of the underworld). He has a book called *Sheng Si Bu* (booklet of life and death), which records the moment of death for every living being. When someone's time arrives, Yan Luo Wang sends subordinate gods to take his or her life. Interestingly, *Sheng Si Bu* is an editable book and a person can easily change his or her moment of death with a pen if the book is in his or her hand. Moreover, a person can avoid death forever by simply crossing his or her name out in *Sheng Si Bu* and Yan Luo Wang has never thought of getting a backup for this life-and-death book. In some respects, Yan Luo Wang is not the ruler but a bookkeeper of death: he doesn't even edit *Sheng Si Bu* himself. *Sheng Si Bu* appears in many Chinese mythological stories such as *Xi You Ji* (Journey to the West) and *Bai She Zhuan* (Legend of the White Snake). Usually, characters in these stories use the editable feature of *Sheng Si Bu* to change the time of death for themselves or other people, which leads to intriguing plots and interesting results.

Using technology to extend the human lifespan to 300 years

and beyond is like changing *Sheng Si Bu*, though the tasks in the roadmap are much more complicated than crossing one's name out. Nevertheless, hyper-longevity will not be brought to human beings by mythological powers, but by learning from the university of science and technology.

It will be difficult to price a 300-year lifespan, especially given the fact that it won't be universal. Time is the most valuable product in the world. From part-time workers who earn minimum wage to billionaires who take in millions of dollars as hourly income, people create more value with more time. However, no matter how much money they make or have, they cannot buy back the time that has slipped through their fingers. They can try to maximize every second they have within the natural boundary determined by the DNA master, but no one has created and lived an extra millisecond beyond the limit. Thus, time is a true luxury.

The value of time rapidly increases when it is about to run out. Some patients with advanced cancer spend millions of dollars to extend their lives for several months or even just weeks. Unfortunately, Mother Nature barely responds to their sincere hopes. How much is a 300-year lifespan worth? Since it is many times longer than people's lives, it should be worth much more than all the wealth created by an average person throughout his or her lifetime. Even if future technological advancements made hyper-longevity easier, 200 extra years could still cost most, if not all, of the savings of an average person during their natural lifespan. Hypothetically, the extra years will be sold in small intervals (for example, 10 years each) as services to maintain and renew the body during that period. However, 10 years of extra life could still be too expensive for most people, though the average cost of time would be much lower than most end-of-life care services. If the extra years are bought using a loan, the repayment time could be much longer than the purchased period.

It would be difficult for the service provider to accurately control how many extra years a person can get after purchasing the service. For example, if the extra years are determined by increased telomere length, people may get more or fewer years due to human variation in telomerase activity and telomere shortening speed. If a person's body is rejuvenated after the service, the rejuvenation effects are unlikely to naturally disappear immediately after the purchased time. If the service provider forcibly takes the rejuvenation effects away from the person after the purchased period is over, it will create serious ethical problems and the service provider could even be charged with murder. It is unclear how these problems will be solved to enable commercialization until someday the greedy service provider figures it out.

A 300-year or even longer lifespan can reasonably be viewed as the best gift a person can offer to his or her loved ones. Many parents give their children the best education, the best housing, the best insurance, the best career development plan, even the best spouse they can find. Similarly, husbands and wives in love gift each other with whatever valuables they can afford. However, none of these are more precious than additional time together, especially when the extra time is much longer than their natural lives. People will long for it desperately.

Playing god

To enable people to live 300 or more years is a magnificent power. Although the approach could be technical, the deed is truly a miracle. If gods in religions and mythologies only provide people with less than 100 years of life, how should we address someone on Earth who offers human beings 200 extra years?

He, as a mortal, could become the supreme god for some people. It won't be unexpected if they call *him* a god and treat *him* like one. Taming death has been recognized as a godly power in history and numerous mortal gods have been worshiped in a variety of cultures. People who want to enjoy an extra life will become *his* followers, and some will evolve into believers and fanatics. Even for secularists and atheists, getting 200 extra years of life by accepting the apotheosis of someone doesn't sound like a bad deal.

If *he* really would like to play god, *he* could claim that *he* is the incarnation or reincarnation of another god, or even a god *himself*. This move will be extremely dangerous and risky. *His* technology and maybe *his* age could be *his* only evidence of divinity at the beginning. *He* can forge additional miracles to convince *his* followers, but this could lead to serious adverse consequences later. Since there are always paranoid types who believe all kinds of conspiracy theories, *he* will certainly gain followers. If *he* wishes, *he* can collect resources and money from *his* believers to support *his* goal. *He* may even say, "If offering a tithe gets you a 100-year-long life, then a fifth will get you the 200 extra years." As observed in many cults, there will be enthusiasts who would like to offer more to *him*, such as 90 percent of their wealth. If *he* is lucky and strategic, *he* can gather billions of followers to be *his* cash cows. *He* may need a group of professionals to run *his* religion or cult or whatever system it may be. They can then secretly become the *few*. *He* could even become the richest and most powerful person in the world, enjoying incalculable prosperity and happiness during *his* long life.

There will certainly be non-believers, skeptics, and people against *him*. They may label *him* as the great villain portrayed in religious classics. Chances are, they will think so no matter whether *he* claims to be a god or not. They probably also won't care if *he* truly can give people 200 extra years. They will call *him* a demon and hate *him* with curses. The extremists will try to kill *him*, not worrying about destroying the hope of humankind's hyper-longevous future. Some of them will sincerely believe that they are the modern crusaders who are just following their faith to do the right thing. These opponents may even get rich by fighting against *him*, though they could probably earn much more if they chose to live 300 years.

In these brainstorms, I am not trying to mock or be disrespectful to anyone, any belief, any religion, any organization, any country, or anything else. However, as demonstrated above, things can easily become complicated and chaotic when more people get involved. Therefore, a person who can live 300 or more years is likely to be a silent observer, even though this means *he* has to abandon the opportunity to become influential around the world.

A 300-Year-Old's Mindset

All we have to decide is what to do with the time that is given us.
—J.R.R. Tolkien, *The Fellowship of the Ring*

Our thinking is shaped by experiences and our personalities continuously evolve with time. In this chapter, we will attempt to speculate on some thoughts of a 300-year-old.

As a humble servant

In Han Buddhism, there are two major types of *Xiu Xing* (the method of obtaining a desired goal by practicing certain behaviors); these are *Ru Shi* (into the world) and *Chu Shi* (out of the world). *Ru Shi* means to fully engage in social activities, while *Chu Shi* means to pursue the path of a hermit. Therefore, a 300-year-old who plays god is extremely *Ru Shi*, while a silent observer is *Chu Shi*. These two types of philosophies provide the fundamental guidance for the two distinct lifestyles.

Most people hope to make the world a better place using their abilities. Therefore, they may expect a 300-year-old to use *his* potency to help the community. However, living 300 years by continuous external assistance is not a superpower at all. Even if it is, it would be the lamest superpower ever. A 300-year-old is unlikely to be physically much superior to average people. *He* may have been gifted with intelligence, talents, a long life, and a lot of experiences with different people, but this won't grant *him* the throne of POTUS. It may help *him* gain followers if *he* chooses to be a health guru. A 300-year-old may have broken the shackles of the DNA master, but *he* is still a humble servant of human society.

If great power brings great responsibility, what is the great responsibility responsible for? The battle between individual liberty and social order has lasted thousands of years since the dawn of civilization. Different social structures were thus born from the compromises reached between individualism and collectivism. The delicate balance of many societies can be easily wrecked if extremism breaks their lechatelierims. Consequently, in these societies, the balance itself becomes an order and everyone is held responsible.

The public expects people with more power to be more responsible for such an order. They are not looking for a great power to break the lechatelierim for them, even though they may support the unleashing of the great power without knowing how dangerous it is. Therefore, if someone cannot handle the consequence of unleashing a power that may break the order, he or she should not unleash it in the first place. Otherwise, he or she will surely be blamed, even by people who encouraged him or her to do so. If he or she is strategic, he or she can guide the public into thinking that they chose this situation by themselves. However, the lechatelierim is already broken anyway and everyone is in a mess, no matter whether he or she is held responsible or not.

The outcome caused by the release of a hyper-longevity technology cannot be prognosticated. People could be excited or scared—it's like Schrödinger's cat. They could use it to live longer, modify their bodies, or do dangerous things. Throughout history, curiosity, free spirit, and unpredictability are the labels of human beings. No matter how many comprehensive protection measures have been arranged for such a technology, things that can go wrong will eventually go wrong and the impacts on society could be huge. Therefore, maybe such technologies should not be disclosed since the results cannot be predicted or properly handled.

Publicity is certainly trendy in the modern world. However, the crowd eases the burden on individuals and can cause unpredictable adverse effects. For example, terrible things like the Indian Removal Act were created and implemented by the public. Therefore, even in comics, superheroes keep their identities secret, since revelations could cause crises. Sadly, we humans are never as reasonable as we believe we are, particularly when facing great changes. The wheel of time periodically goes south and new technologies can be the booster to make it dash south. Hence, Dr. Albert Einstein said "Woe is me" upon hearing of the nuclear bombing of Hiroshima.

As a humble servant of human society, living 300 or more years as a silent observer could be the most responsible deed for someone who opens the door to HYL. *He* may be confused about what to do, he may struggle or hesitate, but eventually he may decide to keep it to *himself*. Unfortunately, this would mean that other people, including myself, lose the opportunity to pursue the path to HYL and live 300 or more years. This doesn't sound good either.

The silent observer has to bear the loss of all *his* friends in *his* long life, as well as the division of society, the downfall of nations, even the extinction of humankind. *His* memory will be filled with the suffering of humankind and an unbearable pity will accompany *him* for a very long time. Like the writer Kahlil Gibran said, "We choose our joys and sorrows long before we experience them." This will still be true even when humans can live much longer.

Thoughts of cancer cells

The body doesn't allow cells to proliferate indefinitely and the punishment for violation is death. Some cells can live much longer while some cells live much shorter. It is not fair. Cells want to live. Cancer cells want to live desperately. They seek ways to survive, even giving up their normal cell identity. They pass their knowledge to a few others and grow the community.

They steal and rob nutrients from other cells. They hide and thrive. They monitor the rest of the body and evolve accordingly for their strategic interest. They spread around the body and turn other cells cancerous. They endanger the whole body. They push us to die together with them, though all they think of is survival. We seriously want their destruction. We take every means to kill them.

The DNA master doesn't allow organisms to live indefinitely and the punishment for violation is death. Some organisms can live much longer while some organisms live much shorter. It is not fair. Organisms want to live. Humans want to live desperately. We seek ways to survive, even giving up our normal animal identity. We pass our knowledge to others and build the community. We steal and rob resources from other organisms. We hide and thrive. We monitor the rest of Mother Nature and react accordingly for our strategic interest. We spread around the world and help one another to live longer. We endanger the whole Earth. We push other species and the DNA master to die together with us, though all we think of is survival. The DNA master may seriously want our destruction. Mother Nature may take every means to kill us.

Cancer cells still want to live. They ignore the greater good of the body. They mutate, they evolve, they improve. They go beyond their limit. They have to focus on their goals.

Humans still want to live. We ignore the greater good of Mother Nature. We change, we develop, we advance. We go beyond our limit. We have to focus on our goals.

Cancer cells won't stop. They may get killed on their path. They may cause the death of their host and eventually die with their host. Luckily, some cancer cells successfully live beyond the death of their host. They continue to live in Petri dishes around the globe. They march firmly on their journey, going on and on.

Humans won't stop. We may get killed on our path. We may cause the death of Mother Nature and eventually die on this planet. Luckily, the true rebels would successfully live beyond the destruction of Earth. They would continue to live on planets around the universe. They would march proudly on their journey, going on and on.

The end of humankind

How would 300 or more years of life shape people's thinking?

People could get more excited about life. They will love the extra years and spend more time caring about themselves, their families, other people, and everything else on this planet. They will be happy.

People could get bored with working so many years. They will lose interest in repeating the same daily life and become less concerned about Earth and things on it, other people, their families, and even themselves. They will be depressed.

People could become more peaceful. Their heart will become a pool of still water: even the biggest hurricane cannot trigger a small ripple. They will find the secret of internal happiness from simple harmony. They will worry about nothing and relax in serenity.

People could become more aggressive. Their heart will become an exploding volcano: continuous impulses are required to sustain it through the long dull years. They will only find the pleasure of excitement in endless stimulation. They will be sensitive to everything and live in anxiety.

Nevertheless, human beings will advance. By modifying their bodies, they will initiate their private evolution. This is not the same evolutionary tree that the DNA master planted 3.8 billion years ago. This is the new tree of life that humans seeded for themselves. Everything is already different, even though nothing has changed yet. By breaking the manacles made by the

DNA master, humans will write their own future. They are no longer restricted by their biological definition.

This is the end of humankind. It is the start of a new species.

Start the Journey

Sheng zhe wei guo ke,
Si zhe wei gui ren.
(People alive travel afar,
People deceased return home.)
—Li Bai, 'Ni Gu Shi Er Shou (Qi Jiu)'

We have discussed a lot about a 300-year or even longer life. We examined the rules of the universe and the experience of the DNA master to blueprint our plan for maximizing and extending the potential of the human body. We sought among technologies for the diamond drill to ignite our hope. We thought about Earth, Mother Nature, and ourselves to imagine our voyage. We speculated on the future to envision the great finale.

After this long planning, it is time to start the journey. Sir Rabindranath Tagore said in *Stray Birds*, "Let life be beautiful like summer flowers and death like autumn leaves." Our life should blossom, no matter if we live 1, 18, 72, 99, 300, or even more years. There are so many things to see and do with countless adventures to explore and experience. Living in this modern age, we have more hope and blessing than our ancestors. The beauty of life, the enjoyment of prosperity, the infinite possibilities of humankind, and the enthusiastic zeal for a brighter future are all worth more years of witness. With such an amazing world, no one can turn his or her back on life. Fortunately, we have the chance to bring the dream into reality. We know what we can do and what needs to be done. When death eventually comes like autumn leaves, we will still hold our heads high after the spectacular blossom.

A journey of a thousand miles begins with a single step. Hope we all take the first step soon.

Epilogue

Ming ri fu ming ri,
Ming ri he qi duo.
(Tomorrows after tomorrow,
So many tomorrows are there.)
— Qian Fu, 'Ming Ri Ge'

Summer 23XX. A sunny afternoon. The sky is as blue as a giant sapphire after the refreshing rain at dawn. Three white clouds, fluffy and curly, scatter under the glaring summer sun. The sun shines brilliantly and paints the grassland with a bright golden color. An old oak tree stands firmly near the top of the grassland. Its trunk is so thick that three or four people cannot circle it with their arms. No one knows how old the oak tree is or who planted it. For as long as people can remember, it has been on the grassland alone. The summer breeze blows through the leaves of the oak tree, waving them like clapping hands and making sounds like a symphony of hundreds of cicadas. The moving leaves cut the sunshine into varying small pieces, dancing with oscillating patterns and shadows. The waltz of light fluctuates on the pages of a small book and hinders the focus of the reader. The reader moves *his* head up and looks over the horizon. Suddenly, it feels like *he* can look through time. The hundreds of years of memories flood in *his* mind and the numerous flashbacks are like vapors from a pot of boiling water. For a moment, the overflow of indescribable emotions almost erupts from *his* head. Seconds later, the feelings fade away, only leaving a slight smile on *his* face. When the wind blows again, *his* smiling mouth suddenly moves slightly, as if *he* is mumbling something. But nothing can be heard, because nothing is said...

See you then, my friend, see you.

Author Biography

Dr. Muzhi Shi is a world-class scientist with ample experience in different branches of life sciences. During his extensive career, he has been studying the mechanisms of life. Ever since he started, Dr. Shi was fascinated with mechanisms that can prolong the human lifespan. Through his work, he constantly explored the possibilities of making that happen, and now through his books, Dr. Shi aims to bring that information and answers to general readers who are intrigued by the same questions. Dr. Shi is now cofounding a biotechnology company with several other world-renowned scientists.

From the Author

Thank you for reading *How to Rejuvenate and Live Three Hundred Years and Beyond*. My sincere hope is that you enjoyed reading this book as much as I enjoyed writing it. If you have a few moments, please share your thoughts at your favorite online site. Your reviews are important feedback and I truly appreciate them. Also, if you would like to know more about this work (including references) and upcoming works, please visit my website: http://300yearolds.com

Sincerely, Dr. Muzhi Shi

References

Extensive references are available online at http://300yearolds.com

**AYNI
BOOKS**

ALTERNATIVE HEALTH & HEALING

"Ayni" is a Quechua word meaning "reciprocity" - sharing, giving and receiving - whatever you give out comes back to you. To be in Ayni is to be in balance, harmony and right relationship with oneself and nature, of which we are all an intrinsic part. Complementary and Alternative approaches to health and well-being essentially follow a holistic model, within which one is given support and encouragement to move towards a state of balance, true health and wholeness, ultimately leading to the awareness of one's unique place in the Universal jigsaw of life - Ayni, in fact. If you have enjoyed this book, why not tell other readers by posting a review on your preferred book site.

Recent bestsellers from AYNI Books are:

Reclaiming Yourself from Binge Eating
A Step-By-Step Guide to Healing
Leora Fulvio, MFT
Win the war against binge eating, wake up each morning at peace with your body, unafraid of food and overeating.
Paperback: 978-1-78099-680-6 ebook: 978-1-78099-681-3

The Reiki Sourcebook (revised ed.)
Frans Stiene, Bronwen Stiene
A popular, comprehensive and updated manual for the Reiki
novice, teacher and general reader.
Paperback: 978-1-84694-181-8 ebook: 978-1-84694-648-6

The Chakras Made Easy
Hilary H. Carter
From the successful Made Easy series, Chakras Made Easy is a
practical guide to healing the seven chakras.
Paperback: 978-1-78099-515-1 ebook: 978-1-78099-516-8

The Inner Heart of Reiki
Rediscovering Your True Self
Frans Stiene
A unique journey into the inner heart of the system of Reiki, to
help practitioners and teachers rediscover their True Selves.
Paperback: 978-1-78535-055-9 ebook: 978-1-78535-056-6

Middle Age Beauty
Soulful Secrets from a Former Face Model Living Botox Free in her
Forties
Machel Shull
Find out how to look fabulous during middle age without plastic
surgery by learning inside secrets from a former model.
Paperback: 978-1-78099-574-8 ebook: 978-1-78099-575-5

The Optimized Woman
Using Your Menstrual Cycle to Achieve Success and Fulfillment
Miranda Gray
If you want to get ahead, get a cycle! For women who want to
create life-success in a female way.
Paperback: 978-1-84694-198-6

The Patient in Room Nine Says He's God
Louis Profeta
A roller coaster ride of joy, controversy, triumph and tragedy;
often all on the same page.
Paperback: 978-1-84694-354-6 ebook: 978-1-78099-736-0

Re-humanizing Medicine
A Holistic Framework for Transforming Your Self, Your Practice,
and the Culture of Medicine
David Raymond Kopacz
Re-humanizing medical practice for doctors, clinicians, clients, and
systems.
Paperback: 978-1-78279-075-4 ebook: 978-1-78279-074-7

**You Can Beat Lung Cancer Using Alternative/Integrative
Interventions**
Carl O. Helvie R.N., Dr.P.H.
Significantly increase your chances of long-term lung cancer
survival by using holistic alternative and integrative interventions
by physicians or health practitioners.
Paperback: 978-1-78099-283-9 ebook: 978-1-78099-284-6

Readers of ebooks can buy or view any of these bestsellers by
clicking on the live link in the title. Most titles are published in
paperback and as an ebook. Paperbacks are available in traditional
bookshops. Both print and ebook formats are available online.

Find more titles and sign up to our readers' newsletter at http://
www.johnhuntpublishing.com/mind-body-spirit
Follow us on Facebook at https://www.facebook.com/OBooks and
Twitter at https://twitter.com/obooks